ONE STOP DOC

Nervous System

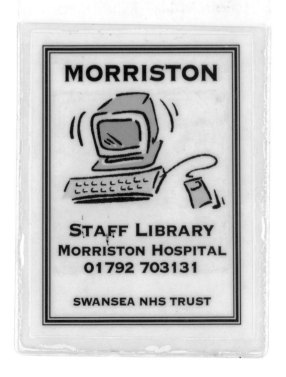

One Stop Doc

Titles in the series include:

Cell and Molecular Biology – Desikan Rangarajan & David Shaw
Editorial Advisor – Barbara Moreland

Gastrointestinal System – Miruna Canagaratnam
Editorial Advisor – Richard Naftalin

Cardiovascular System – Jonathan Aron
Editorial Advisor – Jeremy Ward

Coming soon...

Respiratory System – Jo Dartnell and Michelle Ramsay
Editorial Advisor – John Rees

Musculoskeletal System – Bassel Zebian and Wayne Lam
Editorial Advisor – Alistair Hunter

Renal System and Electrolyte Balance – Panos Stamoulos and Spyros Bakalis
Editorial Advisor – Richard Naftalin and Alistair Hunter

Endocrine and Reproductive Systems – Caroline Jewel and Alexandra Tillett
Editorial Advisor – Stuart Milligan

Nutrition and Metabolism – Miruna Canagaratnam and David Shaw
Editorial Advisor – Barbara Moreland and Richard Naftalin

ONE STOP DOC
Nervous System

Elliott Smock BSc(Hons)
Fifth year medical student, Guy's, King's and
St Thomas' Medical School, London, UK

Editorial Advisor: Clive Coen BA MA DPHIL (OXFORD)
Professor of Neuroscience, Guy's, King's and
St Thomas' Medical School, London, UK

Series Editor: Elliott Smock BSc(Hons)
Fifth year medical student, Guy's, King's and
St Thomas' Medical School, London, UK

ARNOLD

A member of the Hodder Headline Group
LONDON

First published in Great Britain in 2004 by
Arnold, a member of the Hodder Headline Group,
338 Euston Road, London NW1 3BH

http://www.arnoldpublishers.com

Distributed in the United States of America by
Oxford University Press Inc.,
198 Madison Avenue, New York, NY10016
Oxford is a registered trademark of Oxford University Press

Whilst the advice and information in this book are believed to be true and
accurate at the date of going to press, neither the author nor the publisher
can accept any legal responsibility or liability for any errors or omissions
that may be made. In particular (but without limiting the generality of the
preceding disclaimer) every effort has been made to check drug dosages;
however it is still possible that errors have been missed. Furthermore,
dosage schedules are constantly being revised and new side-effects
recognized. For these reasons the reader is strongly urged to consult the
drug companies' printed instructions before administering any of the drugs
recommended in this book.

British Library Cataloguing in Publication Data
A catalogue record for this book is available from the British Library

Library of Congress Cataloging-in-Publication Data
A catalog record for this book is available from the Library of Congress

ISBN 0 340 812494

1 2 3 4 5 6 7 8 9 10

Commissioning Editor: Georgina Bentliff
Project Editor: Heather Smith
Production Controller: Lindsay Smith
Cover Design: Amina Dudhia
Indexer: Indexing Specialists (UK) Ltd

Typeset in 10/12pt Adobe Garamond/Akzidenz GroteskBE by Servis Filmsetting Ltd, Manchester
Printed and bound in Spain

Hodder Headline's policy is to use papers that are natural, renewable and recyclable products
and made from wood grown in sustainable forests. The logging and manufacturing processes
are expected to conform to the environmental regulations of the country of origin.

What do you think about this book? Or any other Arnold title?
Please send your comments to **feedback.arnold@hodder.co.uk**

CONTENTS

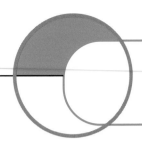

PREFACE

From the Series Editor, Elliott Smock

Are you ready to face your looming exams? If you have done loads of work, then congratulations; we hope this opportunity to practice SAQs, EMQs, MCQs and Problem-based Questions on every part of the core curriculum will help you consolidate what you've learnt and improve your exam technique. If you don't feel ready, don't panic – the One Stop Doc series has all the answers you need to catch up and pass.

There are only a limited number of questions an examiner can throw at a beleaguered student and this text can turn that to your advantage. By getting straight into the heart of the core questions that come up year after year and by giving you the model answers you need this book will arm you with the knowledge to succeed in your exams. Broken down into logical sections, you can learn all the important facts you need to pass without having to wade through tons of different textbooks when you simply don't have the time. All questions presented here are 'core'; those of the highest importance have been highlighted to allow even sharper focus if time for

revision is running out. In addition, to allow you to organize your revision efficiently, questions have been grouped by topic, with answers supported by detailed integrated explanations.

On behalf of all the One Stop Doc authors I wish you the very best of luck in your exams and hope these books serve you well!

From the Author, Elliott Smock

This book has all the absolutely vital information and understanding that you will need to pass an exam on 'The Nervous System'.

Neuroscience has terrified generations of students for decades! Actually, it is a very straightforward and logical subject – however, it is also a very diverse subject and one of the problems is getting to grips with the large knowledge base required to do well.

In this book vision has a large amount of space devoted to it as this is always a hot topic in the exam and a good understanding of it will get you some very easy marks.

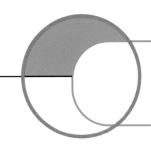

ABBREVIATIONS

ACh	acetylcholine
ACTH	adenocorticotrophic hormone
ADH	antidiuretic hormone
ADP	adenosine diphosphate
AMPA	alpha-amino-3-hydroxy-5-methylisoxazole-4-propionate
ANS	autonomic nervous system
ATP	adenosine triphosphate
BNF	British National Formulary
Ca^{2+}	calcium ion
cAMP	cyclic adenosine monophosphate
cGMP	cyclic guanosine monophosphate
Cl^-	chloride ion
CNS	central nervous system
CSF	cerebrospinal fluid
CVA	cerebrovascular accident
ECG	electrocardiogram
EEG	electroencephalogram
EPP	endplate potential
EPSP	excitatory postsynaptic potential
5-HT	5-hydroxytryptamine
FSH	follicle stimulating hormone
GABA	gamma-aminobutyric acid
HIV	human immunodeficiency virus
iGluR	ionotropic glutamate receptor
IPSP	inhibitory postsynaptic potential
IQ	intelligence quotient
K^+	potassium ion
KCl	potassium chloride
LGN	lateral geniculate nucleus
LH	luteinising hormone
MAO	monoamine oxidase
MCQ	multiple choice question
Mg^{2+}	magnesium ion
mGluR	metabotropic glutamate receptor
MGN	medial geniculate nucleus
MRI	magnetic resonance imaging
Na^+	sodium ion
NMDA	N-methyl-d-aspartate
NO	nitric oxide
NRM	nucleus raphe magnus
NRPG	nucleus reticularis paragiganticellularis
NTD	neural tube defect
PAG	periaqueductal grey
PNS	peripheral nervous system
REM	rapid eye movement
RNA	ribonucleic acid
SHO	senior house officer
SSRI	serotonin selective reuptake inhibitor
TSH	thyroid stimulating hormone
VPL	ventral posterolateral nucleus

SECTION 1

CELLS AND MOLECULES OF THE NERVOUS SYSTEM

CELLS AND MOLECULES OF THE NERVOUS SYSTEM

1. Neuroglial cells

a. Are especially fast conductors of nerve signals
b. Rarely neighbour neurons in the nervous system
c. Include oligodendrocytes and Schwann cells
d. Are neuronal in nature
e. Are all closely related morphologically to neurons

2. Answer true or false to the following

a. Neuroglial cells are usually only found in the CNS
b. Microglial cells contain glial acidic protein
c. Neuroglial cells are essential components of the nervous system
d. Neuroglial cells may contribute to the structure of myelin
e. Neuroglial cells grow in response to injury

3. Match the cell type given in the numbered list with the function below

Options

A. Have an important regulatory role in the central nervous system (CNS)
B. Form myelin in the CNS
C. Modify the composition of cerebrospinal fluid (CSF)
D. Mainly act as scavengers in the CNS
E. Are unable to divide in adult mammals

1. Oligodendrocytes
3. Astrocytes
5. Choroid epithelial cells

2. Neurons
4. Microglia

4. Consider neuroglial cells

a. Schwann cells form myelin in the spinal cord
b. The choroid plexus includes ependymal cells
c. Astrocytes may be found in both white and grey matter
d. Microglia are the main antigen-presenting cells in the CNS
e. Oligodendrocytes store and release neurotransmitters

CNS, central nervous system; CSF, cerebrospinal fluid; K$^+$, potassium ion; PNS, peripheral nervous system

EXPLANATION: NEUROHISTOLOGY (i)

Neuroglial cells are not nerve cells, but are intimately related with neurons and play **important structural and regulatory** roles in the nervous system. They do not conduct nerve signals and have little in common structurally with neurons. Only the Schwann cell is found in the PNS – the rest are found in the CNS. There are five main classes of glial cell:

• Schwann cells
• Astrocytes
• Oligodendrocytes
• Ependymal cells
• Microglial cells

Astrocytes have many important roles in the CNS – their processes often surround the basal lamina of blood vessels and contribute to the formation of the **blood–brain barrier**; during development astrocyte precursors help **guide growing axons**, they provide **structural support** within the CNS, **inactivate neurotransmitters** by uptake and subsequent metabolism and are involved in repair. Astrocytes contain fine filaments made of a substance called **glial fibrillary acid protein**. They may also engulf **neuronal debris**, although this role is mainly carried out by **microglia**.

Astrocytes are responsible for:

1. Supporting framework
2. Formation of the blood–brain barrier
3. Removal of extracellular neurotransmitters
4. Uptake of K^+
5. Guidance for developing nerves
6. Antigen presentation

Oligodendrocytes occur as satellite cells around neurons in the CNS – they are also responsible for **myelination** of axons in the CNS. **Ependymal cells** line the ventricles of the brain. The surfaces of most of these cells are covered with cilia which may aid movement of **CSF** through the ventricular system. Choroid epithelial cells are a type of ependymal cell that cover the surfaces of the **choroid plexus**, modifying the composition of CSF which is secreted. Neurons do not divide in adult mammals and therefore the capacity for brain repair after damage is limited, however some amphibians, such as newts and salamanders, can regenerate whole functional limbs.

Answers
1. F F T F F
2. F F T T T
3. 1 – B; 2 – E; 3 – A; 4 – D; 5 – C
4. F T T T F

5. Astrocytes

a. Form part of the blood–brain barrier
b. Are found in both white and grey matter
c. Are excitable
d. Take up and store neurotransmitters
e. Form myelin

6. Consider the electron micrograph of part of a neuronal cell body below

Label structures A, B, C and D.
What is the synthetic product of
C? What gross structure is E part
of?

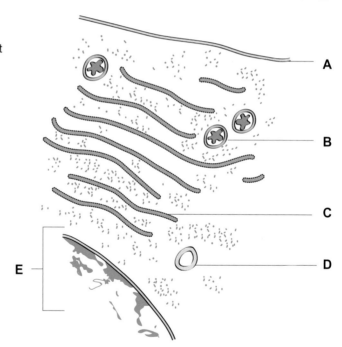

A

B

C

E

D

7. In the study of nerve cells

a. The electron microscope has been of limited use
b. Mitochondria can frequently be seen by light microscope
c. Nissl stains bind to basophilic substances such as RNA and DNA
d. Ramon Cajal was an important pioneer in this field
e. The Golgi body can be viewed under the light microscope with appropriate stains

CNS, central nervous system; RNA, ribonucleic acid

EXPLANATION: NEUROHISTOLOGY (ii)

The electron microscope has been very useful in the study of cell structure. Its high resolution has made it possible to view organelles with great clarity. Most organelles cannot normally be seen under the light microscope – the main exception to this is the nucleus but it sometimes may be seen once it has been stained. The **Golgi body** can also be viewed under the light microscope when stained. Nissl stains are dyes which bind to basophilic (negatively charged) substances such as nucleic acids. Clumps of stained material in the cytoplasm of the cell are termed **Nissl substance** and are actually regions of **rough endoplasmic reticulum** and **ribosomes** associated with RNA. Ramon Cajal shared the 1906 Nobel Prize with Camillo Golgi 'in recognition of their work on the nervous system'. Cajal was particularly interested in the fine structure of the nervous system and wrote extensively on the subject.

6A. **Plasma membrane**: it is a double membrane-bounded, semi-permeable structure
6B. **Mitochondria** (in transverse section)
6C. **Rough endoplasmic reticulum**: in this micrograph it bears a resemblance to the Golgi complex but the latter is normally arranged in an elliptical manner and not associated with ribosomes.
6D. **Lysosome**
6E. **The nucleus**: note the electron dense chromatin

Answers
5. T T F T F
6. see explanation
7. F F T T T

8. On the diagram of a neuron below, mark the following

A. Axon hillock
B. Axon terminal
C. Cell body
D. Dendrite
E. Axon
F. At which site might you see myelination?
G. At which site is the action potential generated?
H. Is protein synthesis possible at this site?

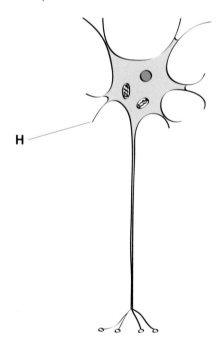

H

9. Neurons in the CNS

a. Have their cell bodies located in the grey matter
b. Have a resting membrane potential of +90 mV
c. Are depolarized to approximately +40 mV on excitation
d. Are always insulated with myelin
e. Are of highly variable morphology

CNS, central nervous system; RNA, ribonucleic acid

EXPLANATION: THE NEURON

Neuron structure is highly variable and specifically related to function – neurons are adapted to whatever job they perform: retinal cells and the hair cells of the auditory system are good examples of specialization. The **resting membrane potential** of a neuron is approximately **−90 mV** – this is a useful value to remember as you may be asked to calculate it in an exam. At its peak the cell membrane is depolarized to about +40 mV.

Concentrated groups of neuronal **cell bodies** make up the **grey matter** of the CNS. **White matter** is made up of **myelinated axonal fibres**. Neurons in the CNS are not always insulated with myelin – some smaller diameter fibres are left bare.

Myelination might be seen at **8E** along the axon and the action potential is generated at **8D** in the axon hillock. Once the **cell body 8C** has been **depolarized** and the change in membrane potential reaches the **axon hillock,** an **action potential** is induced which will propagate along the axon to the terminal **8B**. Protein synthesis has been observed in dendrites **(8H)** – this counters the dogma of protein synthesis only occurring in the cell body. Synapse-associated polyribosome complexes – clusters of polyribosomes bound to mRNA have been identified at these sites and can be seen on electron microscopy.

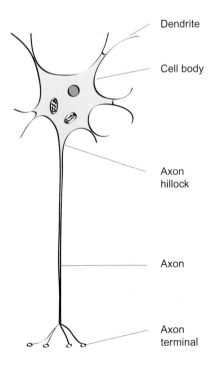

Dendrite

Cell body

Axon hillock

Axon

Axon terminal

Answers
8. See figure and explanation
9. T F T F T

10. Draw and label a typical axo–dendritic synapse. Is the synapse likely to be inhibitory or excitatory?

 11. Complete the numbered statements with the best answer from the following options

Options

A. Monoamine oxidase B
C. Mitochondria
E. In two directions
G. Neurotransmitter reuptake
I. Synaptic vesicles

B. Gap junctions
D. One way only
F. Neurotransmitters
H. Neurotransmitter synthesis
J. Receptors

1. Nerve impulses are transmitted ......
2. In a chemical synapse signal transmission is mediated by ......
3. Receptor activation may be terminated by ......
4. The surface of the postsynaptic membrane contains ......
5. Neurotransmitters are stored in ......

12. The transmission of an action potential in motor neurons usually takes the following route

a. Dendrite → cell body → synapse → axon terminal
b. Cell body → dendrite → axon terminal → synapse
c. Synapse → axon terminal → cell body → dendrite
d. Axon hillock → axon → synapse
e. Axon terminal → synapse → dendrite → cell body

13. Consider chemical synapses

a. Neurotransmission is bidirectional
b. Termination of a signal is by enzyme breakdown only
c. Neurotransmitter release is via endocytosis
d. Voltage-gated Ca^{2+} channels trigger neurotransmitter release
e. Neurotransmitters are stored in synaptic vesicles

Ca^{2+}, calcium ion

EXPLANATION: NEUROTRANSMISSION AND THE SYNAPSE (i)

Below is a diagram of a typical axo-dendritic synapse.

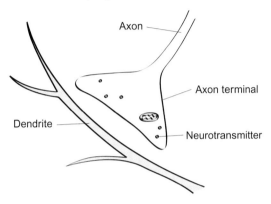

Synapses are structures that permit a neuron in a neuronal circuit to pass information to another cell – either from **neuron to neuron**, or from a **neuron** to another cell type such as a **muscle cell**. There are two main types of synapse: **chemical** – mediated by neurotransmitters or more rarely, **electrical** – mediated by **gap junctions**.

Neurotransmitters are stored in **synaptic vesicles** in the presynaptic terminal. Once released they act on receptors on the surface of the postsynaptic membrane and so act in one direction only. **Activity** in the synapse is terminated by **breakdown of the neurotransmitter** in the synaptic cleft by catabolic enzymes, or by **reuptake** into the presynaptic terminal for recycling.

Synapses on dendrites tend to be **excitatory**, **synapses on cell bodies** are often **inhibitory**. Electrical signals are sent down axons from neuron to target cell by **action potential**.

After an **action potential** is initiated in the **axon hillock** it is transmitted along the **axon** down to an **axon terminal** where the impulse is transmitted across the synapse.

Neurotransmission only proceeds in **one direction** since **synapses** can only send signals one way. Since the neurotransmitter has to diffuse across the synaptic cleft there is a **delay of 0.05 ms** before it reaches its conjugate receptor on the postsynaptic membrane. Once the neurotransmitter has been released it is normally either broken down **enzymatically** at its site of action or removed from the synaptic cleft by being **taken up** into the presynaptic terminal. **Neurotransmitters** are stored in **synaptic vesicles** in the axon terminal: depolarization of the nerve terminal and activation of **voltage-gated Ca^{2+} channels** causes **vesicles** to **fuse** with the axon terminal membrane, releasing the neurotransmitter into the synaptic cleft. This process is termed **exocytosis**.

Answers
10. See figure and explanation
11. 1 – D, 2 – F, 3 – G, 4 – J, 5 – I
12. F F F T F
13. F F F T T

14. Use the options below to complete the statements in the numbered list

Options

A. 2 nm
C. 100 nm
E. gamma-aminobutyric acid (GABA)
G. Glycine
I. Magnesium (Mg^{2+})

B. 20 nm
D. Glutamate
F. Acetylcholine (ACh)
H. Calcium (Ca^{2+})
J. Chloride (Cl$^-$)

1. Synapses are approximately ...... wide
2. Neurotransmitter release from synaptic vesicles is triggered by ......
3. Neurotransmitter release may be inhibited by which the ...... ion
4. Hyperpolarization by GABA is mediated by increased permeability to ......
5. A common example of an excitatory neurotransmitter in the CNS is ......

15. At the synapse

a. Neurotransmitter release usually depends on activation of voltage-gated Ca^{2+} channels
b. The excitatory postsynaptic potential (EPSP) is an all or nothing event
c. A ligand-gated ion channel relies on an electrical stimulus for activation
d. The breakdown of ACh in the synaptic cleft is responsible for the termination of its effect
e. Free Ca^{2+} concentration is greater in the extracellular fluid than the intracellular fluid

16. Draw and label a typical neuromuscular junction

Be sure to label the presynaptic terminal, mitochondria, ACh neurotransmitter, acetylcholinesterase, synaptic cleft, endplate.

ACh, acetylcholine; Ca^{2+}, calcium ion; Cl$^-$, chloride ion; CNS, central nervous system; EPSP, excitatory postsynaptic potential; GABA, gamma-aminobutyric acid; Mg^{2+}, magnesium ion

EXPLANATION: THE SYNAPSE (ii)

In the **chemical synapse** the width of the **synaptic cleft** is approximately **20 nm** (about the width of 200 atoms joined end to end). Depolarization of the **presynaptic terminal** permits Ca^{2+} to enter the cell which **triggers neurotransmitter release**. Mg^{2+} is a divalent ion like Ca^{2+} and has high affinity for the Ca^{2+} receptor, but low efficacy (it cannot activate the receptor). One action of GABA ion channels is to permit entry of negatively charged **Cl^- ions** into the cell which make the interior much more **negative** i.e. the potential is reduced from −70 mV to −90 mV – this is called **hyperpolarization**. **GABA** normally acts as an **inhibitory** neurotransmitter, indeed, this is the most common CNS transmitter. **Excitatory** neurotransmitters have the opposite effect and cause the cell membrane to depolarize – in the CNS, **glutamate** is the most important example of an excitatory neurotransmitter.

The other type of synapse is the **electrical synapse** (gap junction). This permits communication between cells but does not rely on neurotransmitters. Gap junctions are pores made up of protein subunits called **connexons** and permit free passage of many small molecules, but most importantly ions. The distance they travel through the plasma membrane is very small – approximately **2 nm**. Groups of cells joined by gap junctions are known as a **syncitium** and allow signals to be sent through cells as an electrical wave – an example of tissue with a syncitium of gap junctions is smooth muscle in the gut and cardiac muscle.

A typical chemical synapse is activated in the following way: Ca^{2+} enters the **presynaptic terminal** through voltage-operated Ca^{2+} channels – this is the normal stimulus for neurotransmitter release. Some drugs like **reserpine** may cause discharge of the contents of synaptic vesicles (in the case of reserpine the vesicles contain noradrenaline and serotonin), bypassing the usual pharmacological release route. The **EPSP** is produced by activation of ligand-gated ion channels on the postsynaptic membrane. Its magnitude depends on the number of ion channels activated but in theory even a single activated channel could produce an EPSP; however, this would not be strong enough to develop a postsynaptic action potential. **Ligand-gated** channels require ligands (molecules) for their activation. ACh is broken down in the synaptic cleft by **acetylcholinesterase** and is taken up into the presynaptic terminal. Ca^{2+} relies on a diffusion gradient to enter the presynaptic terminal so its concentration must be higher outside.

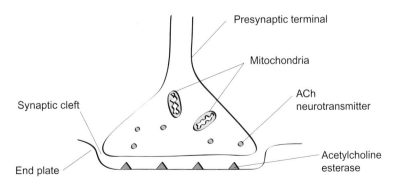

17. At the neuromuscular junction synaptic vesicles contain

   a. ADP
   b. ATP
   c. Acetylcholine (ACh)
   d. Ca^{2+}
   e. Troponin

18. The neuromuscular junction

   a. Has a postsynaptic endplate
   b. May use dopamine as a neurotransmitter
   c. Relies on Na^+ influx to activate Ca^{2+} channels
   d. Consists of a synapse between a sensory neuron and a muscle cell
   e. Terminates neurotransmitter action only by reuptake

19. Annotate the diagrams below showing how an action potential is transmitted across the synapse

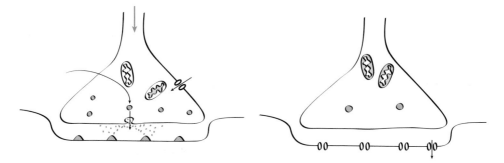

20. The motor unit is defined as

   a. Many myofibrils within the sarcolemma
   b. A motor neuron and the muscle fibres innervated by it
   c. Many motor endplates at the neuromuscular junction
   d. The functional filaments within a muscle fibre
   e. None of the above

ACh, acetylcholine; ADP, adenosine diphosphate; ATP, adenosine triphosphate; cAMP, cyclic AMP; Ca^{2+}, calcium ion; EPP, endplate potential; K^+, potassium ion; Na^+, sodium ion

EXPLANATION: THE NEUROMUSCULAR JUNCTION

An **action potential** travels down the axon of a motor neuron to the **axon terminal**. The **cell membrane** of the axon terminal is **depolarized**. The depolarization activates **voltage-dependent Ca^{2+} channels**. Ca^{2+} **influx** into the axon terminal triggers **release of ACh** stored in secretory vesicles into the synaptic cleft. The ACh binds to **nicotinic ACh receptors** on the postsynaptic membrane, activating them. These ACh receptors are **ligand-gated ion channels** – once activated they permit Na^+ and K^+ to pass through them. The **influx of Na^+** and the **efflux of K^+** depolarizes the postsynaptic membrane (known in the case of the neuromuscular junction as the **endplate**). This creates an **EPP** in the endplate, initiating muscle fibre contraction. ACh in the synaptic cleft is broken down into acetyl and choline by **acetylcholinesterase**

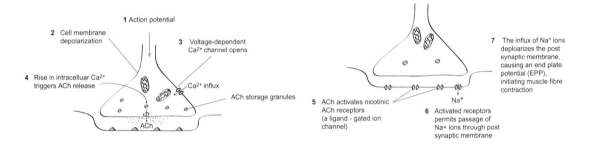

cAMP is not involved in signal transduction at the neuromuscular junction. **Following depolarization the cell membrane is hyperpolarized** and temporarily unresponsive to further stimulation.

A **motor unit** is defined as the collection of muscle fibres supplied by one motor neuron. An example is shown below.

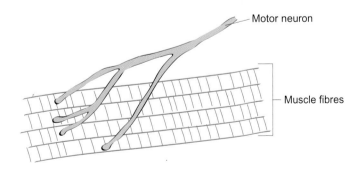

---

21. What are the two main receptor mechanisms seen in pharmacology?

Give examples of those found in the CNS in terms of glutamate receptors and briefly describe their mode of action.

G-protein linked transmembrane receptor in diagrammatic form

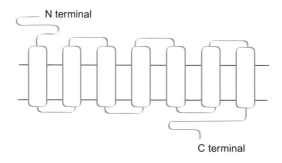

N terminal

C terminal

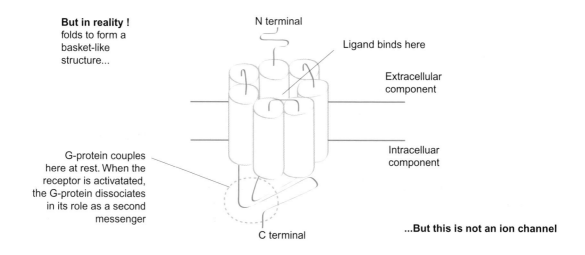

But in reality !
folds to form a
basket-like
structure...

N terminal

Ligand binds here

Extracellular
component

Intracelluar
component

G-protein couples
here at rest. When the
receptor is activatated,
the G-protein dissociates
in its role as a second
messenger

C terminal

...But this is not an ion channel

AMPA, alpha-amino-3-hydroxy-5-methylisoxazole-4-propionate; Ca²⁺, calcium ion; CNS, central nervous system; iGluR, ionotropic glutamate receptor; mGluR, metabotropic glutamate receptor; NMDA, N-methyl-D-aspartate; NO, nitric oxide

EXPLANATION: RECEPTOR MECHANISMS

Glutamate is the major **excitatory neurotransmitter** in the CNS so it is useful to know something about it. The first main groups of receptors are those regulating the activation of ion channels – **ionotropic** or **ligand-gated channel receptors (1)**. The second type are **G-protein-coupled receptors (2)**. Activation of these receptors produces slower effects, typically via a G-protein which in turn may act directly on an ion channel or by a second messenger system.

(1) Ionotropic glutamate receptors are shown below. Ionotropic receptors are **ion channels**. Binding of glutamate to the active site of the iGluR produces one of two types of response:

• **Fast membrane depolarization** lasting approx 1 ms – similar to the action of ACh
• **A distinctly separate membrane depolarization** over an increased time period of 10–15 ms.

There are three subclasses of ionotropic glutamate receptors: the most important are **NMDA receptors** which are Ca^{2+} ion channels. The two other varieties are **AMPA** and **kainate** receptors (non-NMDA receptors).

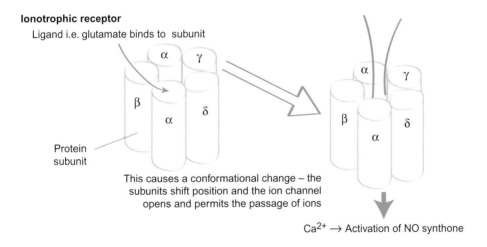

Ionotrophic receptor
Ligand i.e. glutamate binds to subunit

α γ

β δ
α

Protein subunit

This causes a conformational change – the subunits shift position and the ion channel opens and permits the passage of ions

α γ

β δ
α

$Ca^{2+} \rightarrow$ Activation of NO synthone

(2) Metabotropic glutamate receptors are shown in the two figures opposite. These are **G-protein-linked, transmembrane receptors** – to date six varieties have been characterized by cDNA probes and are described as mGluR1–mGluR6. mGluRs are large proteins (850–1150 amino acids) and the tertiary protein structure is made up of seven transmembrane proteins.

22. In pharmacology an antagonist is a drug that

a. Has no affinity for a receptor
b. Blocks the action of a neurotransmitter
c. Has toxic effects
d. Converts excitatory postsynaptic potentials (EPSPs) into inhibitory postsynaptic potentials (IPSPs)
e. Mimics or increases the effect of a neurotransmitter

23. Ionotropic receptors

a. May be permeable to divalent ions
b. Are activated by neuropeptides
c. Are protein structures with seven transmembrane domains
d. Mediate fast inhibitory neurotransmission
e. Mediate fast excitatory neurotransmission

24. Amino acid neurotransmitters

a. Have their cell bodies located in discrete brain nuclei
b. Act exclusively on ionotropic receptors
c. Are released in response to autoreceptor activation
d. Share nerve terminals with other types of neurotransmitter
e. Are broken down only by catabolic enzymes

25. Amino acid neurotransmitters

a. Have both excitatory and inhibitory effects
b. May be involved in long-term potentiation
c. Are thought to play a role in excitotoxic cell death
d. Include glycine which is found in the spinal cord
e. Are not likely to be involved in epilepsy

Ca²⁺ calcium ion; Cl⁻ chloride ion; CNS, central nervous system; EPSP, excitatory postsynaptic potential; GABA, gamma-aminobutyric acid; IPSP, inhibitory postsynaptic potential; NMDA, N-methyl-D-aspartate

EXPLANATION: RECEPTOR PHARMACOLOGY AND NEUROTRANSMITTERS

An **antagonist** has affinity for a receptor, but not **efficacy** – therefore it binds to the receptor but does not activate it, or mimic the effects of the neurotransmitter. By competing with the neurotransmitter for binding sites, the antagonist blocks the effects of the neurotransmitter (agonist). By preventing the effects of an agonist, an antagonist may have toxic effects, but this is not always the case. **EPSPs** are set up in the **postsynaptic membrane** after activation of excitatory receptors in that membrane. **IPSPs** occur in **hyperpolarized regions** in the postsynaptic terminal – the hyperpolarized state of these regions **blocks activation of the nerve fibre** and prevents signals being transmitted along it.

Examples of **amino acid neurotransmitters** are **glutamate** and **glycine**. Their cell bodies are grouped together to form specific nuclei in the CNS – as are other types of neurotransmitter-specific neurons in the brain. Amino acids may have an **excitatory** or an **inhibitory** effect on the CNS. Glutamate acts on **NMDA** receptors which are Ca^{2+} channels and has an **excitatory** effect. It is thought that glutamate may play a role in inducing long-term potentiation – a prolonged excitation of the cell membrane at the synapse – which has been suggested to be a mechanism for memory formation. Glutamate also probably has a role in the excitotoxic death of cells. In stroke or other trauma to the brain, neurons containing glutamate may be ruptured; the excess glutamate spills out in the extracellular space depolarizing surrounding neurons. This intense activity is thought to generate large amounts of toxic free radicals inside the cells which poisons them, causing more cell death. Amino acid neurotransmitters are also implicated in epilepsy. **GABA** (in the CNS) and **glycine** (in the spinal cord) both act on Cl^- channels and have an **inhibitory** effect.

Answers
22. F T F F F
23. T F F T T
24. T F T T F
25. T T T T F

26. Match the neurotransmitters in the numbered list with the correct biochemical class from this list:

Options

A. Inhibitory amino acid
C. Monoamine
E. Peptide

B. Excitatory amino acid
D. Neuropeptide

1. Dopamine
3. Glutamate
5. Glycine

2. Substance P
4. Noradrenaline

27. Match the neurotransmitters in the numbered list with their precursors below

A. alpha-Ketoglutarate
C. Choline
E. Tryptophan

B. Glycine
D. Tyrosine

1. 5-Hydroxytryptamine (5-HT)
3. Dopamine
5. Glutamate

2. Acetylcholine (ACh)
4. Noradrenaline

28. Neurotransmitters

Match the neurological condition in the numbered list with the neurotransmitter MOST likely to be involved in its aetiology or subsequent course

Options

A. Glutamate
C. Dopamine
E. Noradrenaline

B. Acetylcholine (ACh)
D. gamma-aminobutyric acid (GABA)

1. Parkinson's disease
3. Alzheimer's disease
5. Stroke

2. Huntington's chorea
4. Epilepsy

ACh, acetylcholine; GABA, gamma-aminobutyric acid; 5-HT, 5-hydroxytryptamine (serotonin)

EXPLANATION: NEUROTRANSMITTERS AND NEUROLOGICAL DISEASE

The following are **amino acid neurotransmitters**: glutamate (excitatory); gamma-aminobutyric acid (GABA) (inhibitory); glycine (inhibitory). The following are **monamine neurotransmitters**: noradrenaline; dopamine; serotonin (5-HT); histamine. Acetylcholine is a **muscarinic** and **nicotinic** neurotransmitter. The following are **neuropeptide transmitters**: substance P; neuropeptide Y.

Most **amine neurotransmitters** work via **metabotropic** receptors (via G-proteins) but at least one serotonin ionotropic receptor has been identified. Release of these neurotransmitters is self-regulated by feedback on **autoreceptors**. Released neurotransmitters bind to autoreceptors on the presynaptic terminal and cause decreased local synthesis and release of neurotransmitter. More than one type of neurotransmitter can occupy a nerve terminal; this allows 'cotransmission'. **Monoamine** neurotransmitters are taken back up into the presynaptic terminal and broken down by **monoamine oxidase B**.

The synthesis pathways are illustrated below.

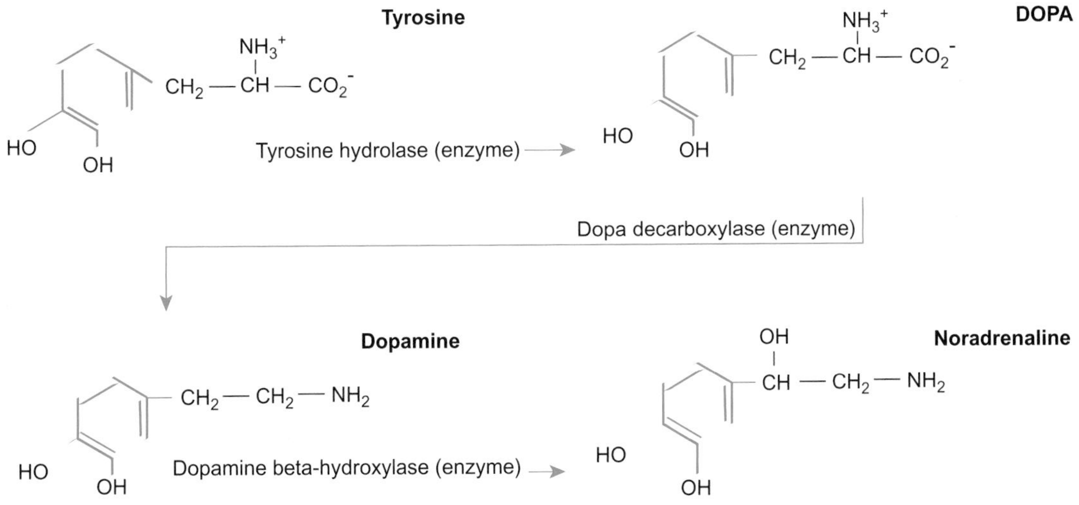

Tyrosine

$CH_2 - \overset{\overset{NH_3^+}{|}}{CH} - CO_2^-$

Tyrosine hydrolase (enzyme) →

DOPA

$CH_2 - \overset{\overset{NH_3^+}{|}}{CH} - CO_2^-$

Dopa decarboxylase (enzyme)

Dopamine

$CH_2 - CH_2 - NH_2$

Dopamine beta-hydroxylase (enzyme) →

Noradrenaline

$\overset{\overset{OH}{|}}{CH} - CH_2 - NH_2$

(in the adrenal glands noradrenaline is converted to adrenaline)

Parkinson's disease is caused by damage to the **nigrostriatal tract** and a subsequent dopamine deficiency. Both **Huntington's chorea** and **Alzheimer's disease** are caused by the loss of **cholinergic neurons**. It has been suggested that underactivity of GABA or overactivity of glutamate channels may be a cause of epilepsy (see page 125 for more information on neurological disorders).

Answers
26. 1 – C, 2 – E, 3 – B, 4 – C, 5 – A
27. 1 – E, 2 – C, 3 – D, 4 – D, 5 – A
28. 1 – C, 2 – B, 3 – B, 4 – A, 5 – A

29. Amphetamine

a. Has been used to treat attention deficit disorder in children
b. Causes release of noradrenaline and adrenaline
c. Can make adults restless
d. Stimulates appetite
e. Does not cause dependence

30. Outline the mechanism of action of amphetamine

31. Hypnotics

a. Are used to treat sleeping disorders
b. May act on GABA receptors
c. Have a relatively long half-life
d. Include benzodiazepines and barbiturates
e. Often have sedative effects

32. Benzodiazepines may cause

a. Respiratory depression
b. Dependence
c. Reduction in muscle tone
d. Reduction in the amount of rapid eye movement (REM) sleep
e. Hangover

33. Neuropharmacology

a. Benzodiazepines act on glutamate receptors
b. Acetylcholinesterase inhibitors increase ACh production
c. Serotonin receptor antagonists promote the firing of 5-hydroxytryptamine (5-HT) neurones
d. The effects of morphine can be reversed by naloxone
e. Amphetamine is a selective beta-adrenergic agonist

ACh, acetylcholine; GABA, gamma-aminobutyric acid; MAO, monoamine oxidase; REM, rapid eye movement; 5-HT, 5-hydroxytryptamine (serotonin)

EXPLANATION: THE PHARMACOLOGICAL MODULATION OF NEUROTRANSMITTERS

Amphetamine is classed as a **sympathomimetic** i.e. it partially or completely mimics the actions of noradrenaline and adrenaline.

Amphetamine closely resembles **noradrenaline** and is taken up into the nerve terminal by the high-affinity transport system (a transmembrane protein), uptake 1, which is normally responsible for the reuptake of noradrenaline from the synaptic cleft. It acts as an indirect sympathomimetic inside the nerve terminal by **displacing vesicular** (stored) **noradrenaline** into the cytoplasm.

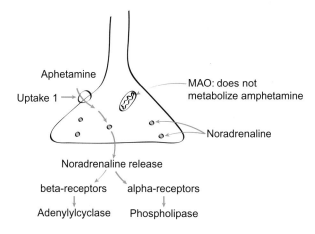

Some of this noradrenaline is metabolized by **MAO**, but the rest is released by carrier-mediated transport to activate adrenoreceptors. **Amphetamine is resistant to MAO**, which potentiates its action in the nerve terminal. Its peripheral actions are **tachycardia** and **hypertension** and its central actions are mediated through the release of catecholamines (30).

34. Use the Nernst equation below to calculate the equilibrium potential of K^+ across a typical mammalian cell membrane.

$$E = \frac{RT}{F} \ln \frac{[K]_o}{[K]_i}$$

F = Faraday's constant = 96 487 C/mol
R = gas constant = 8.314 J/mol/K
T = absolute temperature = 273 K (+ degrees C for mammalian body temperature) = 310 K
$[K]_o$ = extracellular K^+ concentration = 4 mM
$[K]_i$ = intracellular K^+ concentration = 150 mM

35. Intracellular and extracellular fluid

Look at the concentrations of ions in mammalian intra- and extracellular fluid.
A and **B.** Add the values for A and B to the nearest 10 mM.
C. Other than Cl⁻ what class of biochemical is responsible for the bulk of the negative charge in blood and axoplasm?
D. Below is a recording of an action potential from an axon in a solution of different ionic strengths. Which ion is likely to be depleted to produce these effects?

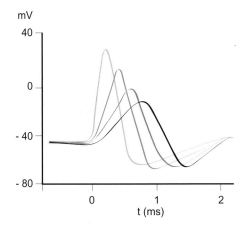

	Intracellular fluid (mM)	Extracellular fluid (mM)
K⁺	A	10
Na⁺	10	120
Cl⁻	B	130

Ca²⁺, calcium ion; Cl⁻, chloride ion; E_k, equilibrium potential; K⁺, potassium ion; KCl, potassium chloride; Na⁺, sodium ion

EXPLANATION: THE NERNST EQUATION AND MEMBRANE PHYSIOLOGY (i)

The Nernst equation allows us to calculate the Equilibrium potential (E_k) for an ion.

To understand the Nernst equation it's a good idea to imagine a model which works in the same way as the **semi-permeable cell membrane** of a **mammalian cell**. Imagine a container divided in half by a **semi-permeable membrane** – in this case **permeable only to K^+ ions**. We can put a strong concentration of KCl in one compartment (to simulate the levels of K^+ in a cell, $[K]_i$) and a weaker concentration in the other (to simulate the levels of K^+ outside the cell, $[K]_o$). A **concentration gradient** exists between the strong and weak solutions, but **only the K^+ ions can move across the barrier**. The movement of the positively charged K^+ ions down the **concentration gradient upsets the balance of the charges in both compartments** – the 'strong solution compartment' becomes more **negatively** charged, and the 'weak solution compartment' becomes more **positively** charged. There comes a point when the force generated by the electrical charge across the membrane is **equal and opposite** to the force generated by the concentration gradient and there is **no net movement** of ions across the membrane. We can then say the ions are in a sort of **equilibrium**.

The resulting electrical potential across the membrane (in this case for K^+) is called the **equilibrium potential**.

The Nernst equation can be applied to any ion in equilibrium across a semi-permeable membrane. If the charge on the ion differs from +1 as in the case of K^+ or Na^+, the equation must be adapted to take this into account, using z, the value for ionic charge.

K^+ $z = +1$ Na^+ $z = +1$ Cl^- $z = -1$ Ca^{2+} $z = +2$

So:

$$E_k = \frac{RT}{zF} \ln = \frac{[K]_o}{[K]_i}\ 8.314 \times 310/96{,}487 \times \ln 4/150 = -0.097\ \text{V}\ (-97\ \text{mV})$$

35

A. 130 mM
B. 10 mM

Negatively charged proteins such as albumin are responsible for the bulk of the negative charge in blood and axoplasm (35C) – these are effectively compartmentalized and are **too large** to travel through ion channels. Depletion of Na^+ is likely to produce the effects shown in the figure (35D).

36. In a neuron at −90 mV

    a. Na⁺ and K⁺ ions are in dynamic equilibrium
    b. There is no net movement of K⁺ ions
    c. There is no net movement of cations
    d. There is no net movement of Na⁺ ions
    e. All of the above are correct

37. The resting potential of the cell membrane is largely determined by

    a. Na⁺ ions   **b.** K⁺ ions
    c. Water   **d.** Cl⁻ ions
    e. Ca²⁺ ions

38. Consider the drawing shown of a typical neuronal action potential

    A. To which ion is the cell membrane most permeable here?
    B. To which ion is the cell membrane most permeable here?
    C. What state is the membrane potential at here?
    D. What state is the membrane potential at here?

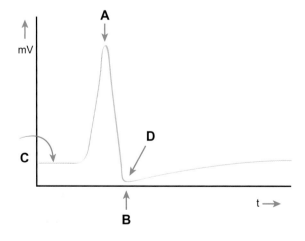

Ca²⁺, calcium ion; Cl⁻, chloride ion; K⁺, potassium ion; Na⁺, sodium ion

EXPLANATION: MEMBRANE PHYSIOLOGY (ii)

When the **cell membrane is at rest**, the ions on either side of the membrane are in **equilibrium** – there is no net movement of ions; however, they do pass across the membrane.

The resting potential of the cell membrane is largely determined by the equilibrium potential of K^+ and is usually around −90 mV. Na^+ also has an effect but it is very small compared to that of K^+. The membrane resting potential is not significantly affected by the equilibrium potential of Cl^- as both values are very similar. Ca^{2+} has little effect as its concentration is so low. Water has no effect as it has no net charge.

Permeability of the cell membrane to Na^+ and K^+ during the generation of an action potential follows the pattern below which is responsible for the distinctive action potential shape. At C the **membrane is at rest** – at this point there is a **balance** between the amounts of Na^+ **and** K^+ **entering and leaving the cell**. The first step in the production of an action potential is a transient **increase in permeability** of the cell membrane to Na^+ which causes the cell membrane to depolarize – the **inside** of the cell becomes more **positively** charged. This is followed shortly afterwards by a transient increase in permeability to K^+, causing the inside of the cell to become more negative than when at rest. The overall effect is that the **inside** of the cell becomes much more **negative**. The increase in permeability to Na^+ and K^+ ions occurs through the activation of voltage-operated ion channels. As their name suggests they are activated at specific voltages – in this case when the cell membrane is depolarized. The changes in permeability to Na^+ and K^+ are shown in the diagram below.

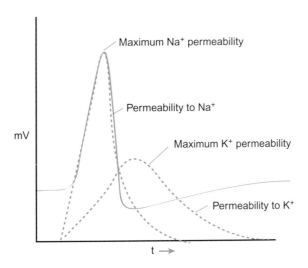

39. Voltage-gated Na$^+$ channels

    a. Also allow passage of K$^+$ ions
    b. Are ion channels
    c. May be activated by acetylcholine (ACh)
    d. Are activated and inactivated by depolarization
    e. Are activated by depolarization and Na$^+$ influx ceases only when the membrane returns to rest

40. Which of the statements below most accurately describes the membrane potential at the peak of an action potential?

    a. Positive – Na$^+$ conductance is greater than that of K$^+$
    b. Positive – K$^+$ conductance is greater than that of Na$^+$
    c. Equal to 0 mV as Na$^+$ and K$^+$ conductance are equal
    d. Negative as this is close to the equilibrium potential for K$^+$
    e. Positive as this is close to the equilibrium potential for K$^+$

41. Hyperpolarization

    a. Is caused by a negative shift in the cell's membrane potential
    b. Is caused by a positive shift in the cell's membrane potential
    c. Occurs in an all-or-none fashion
    d. Can trigger an action potential if large enough
    e. Is frequently triggered by Na$^+$ ions

ACh, acetylcholine; Cl$^-$, chloride ion; K$^+$, potassium ion; Na$^+$, sodium ion

EXPLANATION: MEMBRANE PHYSIOLOGY (iii)

Hyperpolarization occurs when the **inside charge** of the cell becomes a lot more **negative** – more so than when it is simply depolarized. Movement of K^+ **ions out of the cell** or movement of Cl^- **ions into the cell** makes the **inside** more **negative**. If Na^+ ions moved into the cell, the charge inside would become more positive. This extreme negative charge effectively paralyses the Na^+ channels and the cell enters a **refractory stage** where it is unable to be excited again until its membrane charge returns to normal.

42. Myelin

a. Contains a high proportion of lipids
b. Inhibits action potentials in axons
c. Forms sheaths that are interrupted by nodes of Ranvier
d. Fully insulates nerves at birth
e. May be lost in some diseases

43. Saltatory conduction describes:

a. The motion of Na$^+$ ions as they enter the nerve
b. How an action potential jumps from one node to the next
c. How an action potential jumps from axon to axon
d. Transmission of impulses from nerves to Schwann cells
e. Transmission of impulses from nerves to astrocytes

44. Conduction velocity in axons

a. Is constant regardless of axon diameter
b. Is greater in small unmyelinated axons
c. Is greater in large myelinated axons
d. Is generally faster in motor axons than sensory axons
e. Is faster in lower temperatures

45. Consider the neurogram below

The neurogram was recorded from a patch of skin on the arm. An electrical stimulus was applied via an electrode and a recording made from a second electrode 50 cm from the stimulus. Three separate bursts of action potentials were recorded and are shown in the neurogram.

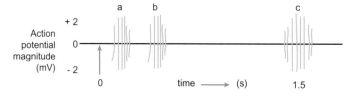

a. The fibres responsible for burst 'a' are solely alpha fibres
b. The fibres responsible for burst 'b' are C fibres
c. Burst 'a' fibres are responsible for the sensation of light touch
d. The fibres responsible for bursts 'b' and 'c' are both likely to be myelinated
e. Burst 'c' fibres are more susceptible to local anaesthetics than burst 'a' fibres

HIV, human immunodeficiency virus; Na$^+$, sodium ion

EXPLANATION: NEURONAL CONDUCTION

Myelin is made when **Schwann cells** or **oligodendrocytes** wrap around an axon to form a multilayered spiral structure which **insulates** the axon. Myelination occurs in most axons with a **diameter greater than 1 μm** and **speeds up transmission** of action potentials. Gaps exist between adjacent Schwann cells called **nodes of Ranvier** – these are areas along the nerve fibre where the axon is **uninsulated**. Because of the insulation, the action potential jumps from node to node – this is known as **saltatory conduction** (from the Latin 'saltere' – to dance – not French as is often quoted) and the action potential is transmitted down the axon jumping from node to node.

At **birth** human axons are **not fully myelinated** and it may take several months before this process is complete. Loss of myelin by disease processes can have a devastating effect on the functioning of the nervous system – the most well known **demyelinating disorder** is **mutiple sclerosis**, but there are others such as **progressive multifocal leukoencephalopathy** and **HIV encephalopathy**.

Nerve fibres are arranged into **groups** according to their **size**. The **larger** the axon **diameter** (providing it is myelinated) the **faster** the conduction velocity. The fibres responsible for burst 'a' are **A fibres** (alpha, beta, gamma and delta fibres), those responsible for burst 'b' are **B fibres** and burst 'c' are **C fibres** (**small diameter unmyelinated nerve fibres**). A and B fibres are both myelinated which goes some way to explaining their fast conduction times. Small, thin fibres are more susceptible to hypoxia and drugs like local anaesthetics.

Factors affecting conduction velocity in axons are:

* Axon diameter: the larger the diameter the faster the conduction velocity
* Myelination: causes an increase in conduction velocity
* Resistance: the greater the resistance the slower the conduction velocity
* Temperature: conduction is slower at low temperatures
* Ion concentrations: conduction may slow down with low ion concentrations

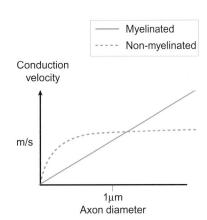

Answers

42. T F T F T
43. F T F F F
44. F F T T F
45. F F F F T

46. Excitatory postsynaptic potentials

a. Usually occur presynaptically
b. May be summated during repetitive presynaptic stimulation
c. Last only for the duration of the presynaptic potential
d. Are an all-or-nothing response to a presynaptic potential
e. Always trigger an action potential

47. Excitatory postsynaptic potentials

a. Are commonly mediated by glutamate
b. Are associated with postsynaptic depolarization
c. May cause a rise in postsynaptic Ca^{2+}
d. Are not summated
e. Activate Cl^- ion channels

48. Inhibitory postsynaptic potentials

a. May be excitatory
b. Are usually triggered by interneurons
c. Play a role in the tendon-jerk reflex
d. May be mediated by GABA or glycine
e. Often inhibit antagonist muscles in reflexes

49. Inhibitory postsynaptic potentials

a. Are additive
b. Cause hyperpolarization
c. Cause an influx of Na^+ ions
d. Cause an influx of Na^+ and Cl^- ions
e. Cause an influx of K^+

ACh, acetylcholine; Ca^{2+}, calcium ion; Cl^-, chloride ion; CNS, central nervous system; EPSP, excitatory postsynaptic potential; GABA, gamma-aminobutyric acid; IPSP, inhibitory postsynaptic potential; K^+, potassium ion; Na^+, sodium ion

EXPLANATION: INHIBITORY AND EXCITATORY POSTSYNAPTIC POTENTIALS

EPSPs occur in the postsynaptic component of neuron–neuron synapses. They are equivalent to the endplate potential in the neuromuscular junction but the neurotransmitter is thought to be **glutamate**, not ACh. The EPSP can trigger an action potential if it is large enough, but may rely on **multiple inputs** from other dendrites which **summate** the EPSPs from various inputs until the required **threshold for depolarization** is reached and an action potential is fired. This is an all-or-nothing response – the magnitude is variable, but only because the separate EPSPs are summated. The EPSP is a relatively long event and typically outlasts the presynaptic potential. Activation of Cl$^-$ channels is associated with inhibition of the postsynaptic terminal and would have the opposite effect to that seen with an EPSP (see explanation of IPSPs below).

As their name suggests, **IPSPs** are inhibitory potentials – they **prevent action potentials** being triggered in the postsynaptic part of the synapse. IPSPs are a useful means of **regulating** neuron function in the CNS by damping down the effects of targeted neurons. A nervous system which could only respond due to excitation would be very clumsy. An IPSP is triggered when an interneuron (in the brain or spinal cord) releases an inhibitory neurotransmitter against the target cell to be inhibited. The **inhibitory neurotransmitter** is often **GABA** or **glycine**. Inhibition occurs through **hyperpolarization** of the target cell's plasma membrane – the GABA opens either Cl$^-$ or K$^+$ channels so either Cl$^-$ enters the cell or K$^+$ leaves it – the end result is the membrane is hyperpolarized which prevents activation.

Whether or not **depolarization** occurs depends on the **balance of EPSPs versus IPSPs**. IPSPs are usually small and act as sinks for the EPSPs.

Answers
46. F T F T F
47. T T T F F
48. F T T T T
49. T T F F T

50. The diagram below shows several stages in the early development of a mammalian embryo

   A. What is the name of the gross structure A?
   B. What does this structure go on to form?
   C. Name the structure at B – of which system is it a precursor?
   D. What is the process called that produces C?

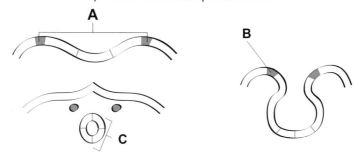

51. Consider neural tube defects

   a. Spina bifida and exomphalos are examples of neural tube defects (NTDs)
   b. Hydrocephalus and lower limb paralysis is an unusual feature of NTDs
   c. NTDs result from failure of the neural tube to fuse
   d. Anencephaly is a fatal condition
   e. Excess folate is a risk factor for NTDs in humans

52. Pair the features in the numbered list with the pathological conditions below

Options

   A. Anencephaly
   C. Myelocele
   E. Meningocele

   B. Spina bifida occulta
   D. Meningomyelocele

   1. The skin, vertebral arches and dura are missing but other meninges are present
   2. Failure of the cranial vault to form
   3. A cyst in the lumbosacral region containing CSF
   4. The severest form of spina bifida with exposed non-functioning neural tissue
   5. A common condition where the skin and the dura around the spinal cord are intact

CNS, central nervous system; CSF, cerebrospinal fluid; NTD, neural tube defect

EXPLANATION: DEVELOPMENT OF THE NERVOUS SYSTEM

The structure at 50A is a neural plate. 50B highlights the neural crest cells – these go on to form the dorsal root ganglia. The structure shown at (C) is the neural tube which is the precursor of the central nervous system (CNS) (50C). The process that forms C is called neurulation (50D).

The **primitive nervous system** starts to form in the **third week** of development when cells of the **dorsal ecto-derm** thicken to form the **neural plate**. The neural plate starts to fold and becomes the **neural groove** – a v-shaped fold. The two side walls are termed **neural folds**; eventually they bend over to meet in the middle and form a tube known as the **neural tube**. The edges join first in the middle, and **close outwards in both directions** with the ends closing last of all. Sometimes the neural folds fail to close correctly resulting in a **neural tube defect** – if the embryo survives it may develop into a fetus with **spina bifida** or **anencephaly**. As the neural plate starts to fold the lateral-most cells migrate outwards – these are **neural crest cells** and are the precursor of the peripheral nervous system. The process of neural tube formation is termed **neurulation** and is the fundamental step in the development of the nervous system.

Sometimes problems occur during development. **Anencephaly** and **spina bifida** result from failure of the neural tube to close correctly during development. **Anencephaly** results from **failure of the neural tube to close anteriorly**, resulting in a fatal brain and skull defect with exposed brain tissue. **Spina bifida** results from **failure of the posterior neural tube to close**; the resulting defect is seen in the lumbosacral region of the spine. Exomphalos is not an example of a NTD – it is a developmental disorder of the gut. **Hydrocephalus** and **paralysis** of varying degrees are common features of spina bifida and depend on the extent of the lesion. **Folate** taken in the first few weeks of pregnancy has been found to prevent a proportion of cases of NTDs – folate-resistant cases are thought to be polygenetic in origin.

The severity of spina bifida varies considerably from the most severe – **myelocele** which is characterized by an open lesion with severely damaged non-functioning spinal cord tissue – through to **spina bifida occulta** in which there is only failure of the vertebral arches to fuse.

Answers
50. See explanation
51. F F T T F
52. 1 – D, 2 – A, 3 – E, 4 – C, 5 – B

STRUCTURE OF THE NERVOUS SYSTEM

STRUCTURE OF THE NERVOUS SYSTEM

1. Consider the brain

a. It consumes 20 per cent of the cardiac output
b. It weighs approximately 1500 g in an adult male
c. It slowly declines in size after 50 years of age
d. It is smaller in the female
e. The size of an individual's brain is related to their intelligence quotient (IQ)

2. Complete the numbered statements from the options given

Options

A. Posterior/superior
B. Anterior/superior
C. Inferior/anterior
D. Posterior/inferior
E. Medial/inferior

In humans the
1. Frontal lobe is ...... to the occipital lobe and ...... to the temporal lobe
2. Temporal lobe is ...... and ...... to the occipital lobe
3. Occipital lobe is ...... and ...... to the parietal lobe
4. Parietal lobe is ...... to the frontal lobe and ...... to the temporal lobe
5. Insula is ...... to the temporal lobe and ...... to the parietal lobe

3. A slice of the cortex where only one hemisphere is visible is likely to be taken in which plane?

a. Sagittal
b. Horizontal
c. Axial
d. Coronal
e. None of the above

EXPLANATION: GROSS STRUCTURE (i)

The brain has high metabolic requirements and thus consumes **20 per cent** of the **cardiac output**. The average weight of an adult **female brain** is approximately **1275 g** – there is no evidence to relate brain size to intelligence in humans. The **male brain** weighs **1500 g**. After the age of 50 years the brain gradually decreases in size but there is not normally any appreciable loss of intellectual ability.

Axial implies a view down the central axis of the nervous system – the other orientations are best described diagramatically:

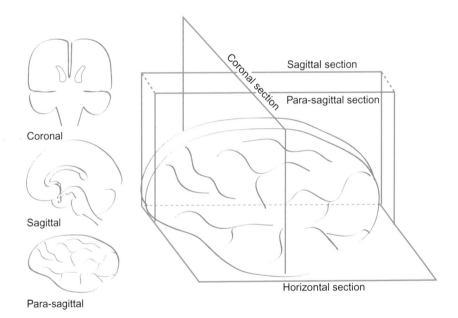

4. Match the structures in the brain in the numbered list with the most appropriate answers below

Options

A. Medulla

B. Diencephalon

C. Cerebrum

D. Midbrain

E. Cerebellum

1. Contains the red nucleus and the substantia nigra
2. Contains the hypothalamus
3. Contains the IX cranial nerve nuclei
4. Contains six cortical layers
5. Contains the dentate nucleus

5. The relations of the corpus striatum

Label the horizontal section through the diencephalon (midbrain) using the numbered list below

1. Corpus callosum
2. Thalamus
3. Pineal gland
4. Genu of the internal capsule
5. Anterior limb of the internal capsule
6. Putamen
7. Head of caudate nucleus
8. Lateral ventricle
9. Corpus striatum
10. Posterior limb of internal capsule
11. Globus pallidus
12. Tail of caudate nucleus

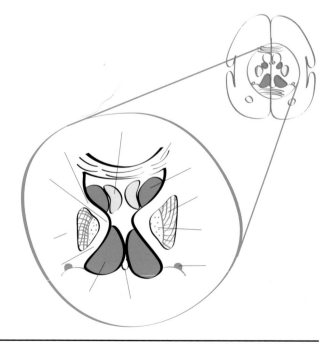

EXPLANATION: GROSS STRUCTURE (ii)

The brain is divided into six functional components. The **medulla**, **pons** and **midbrain** collectively form the **brainstem**. They all contain nerve nuclei, tracts and have regulatory roles which help control basic bodily functions (see pages 47, 53).

1. The **medulla** contains the **olivary nuclei** which project fibres to the cerebellum via the inferior cerebellar peduncles. It also contains **cranial nerve nuclei IX–XII**

2. The **dorsal part of the pons** contains tracts and **cranial nerve nuclei V–XIII**. The **ventral pons** sends fibres to the contralateral cerebellar hemisphere. The pons is connected to the cerebellum by the middle cerebellar peduncles.

3. The **cerebellum** is part of the motor system and helps control posture, balance and co-ordination of movements. It contains the **dentate nuclei.**

4. The **midbrain** contains many interesting parts including the **tectum** (in its roof) which is concerned with the visual and auditory systems. It also includes the motor nuclei – the **red nucleus** and the **substantia nigra** (this is significant in Parkinson's disease see page 127). The midbrain contains **cranial nerve nuclei III–IV** and is connected to the cerebellum by the superior cerebellar peduncles.

5. The **diencephalon** lies at the heart of cerebral hemispheres. It contains the **thalamus** (a mass of nuclei which acts as a relay – receiving incoming information from sensory systems) and the **hypothalamus**, which contains various nuclei (the **hypothalamic nuclei**). The hypothalamus plays an important role in homeostasis (control of blood pressure, temperature) via the autonomic nervous system and releases hormones from the pituitary gland.

6. The cerebrum (telencephalon) is composed of two hemispheres. Each hemisphere is made up of several lobes.

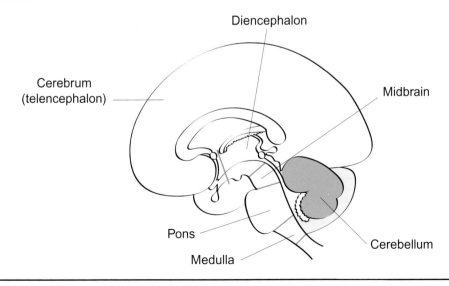

6. The cortical layers of the brain

    a. Usually consist of one layer of cell bodies and one layer of axons
    b. Are not seen in rodents
    c. Are the same thickness throughout the nervous system
    d. Consist of three layers of varying thickness
    e. Consist of six layers of varying thickness

7. Consider the cortical layers of the brain

    a. Brodmann's areas are based on the microscopic structure of the cortical layers
    b. They can be divided into columns
    c. They are more apparent histologically in layers three and five
    d. They are seen throughout the cerebral cortex
    e. They do not include stellate and basket cells

8. On the diagram below, label and briefly state the functions of the parts of the brain labelled A, B, C and D

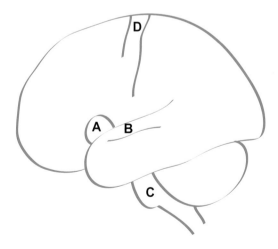

MGN, medial geniculate nucleus

EXPLANATION: THE CEREBRAL CORTEX

The **cerebrum** includes the cerebral cortex, the corpus striatum and the cerebral white matter. The cerebral white matter represents axon tracts in the brain and spinal cord.

The **cerebral cortex** in the human brain has **six cortical layers** which vary in thickness and are seen throughout the brain – they are made up of a variety of cell types including **pyramidal, stellate** and **basket cells**. Brodmann's map of the cerebral cortex was published in 1909 and divided the surface of the cerebral cortex up into 52 small parts – this work was based on the histological arrangement of the cortical layers. Stimulation with microelectrodes has shown that the cells of the cortical layers are arranged in **columns** but these cannot be seen with traditional histological techniques; however, they are important from a functional point of view.

Layers III and V both contain pyramidal cells – their large cell bodies account for the distinctive darker appearance of these layers

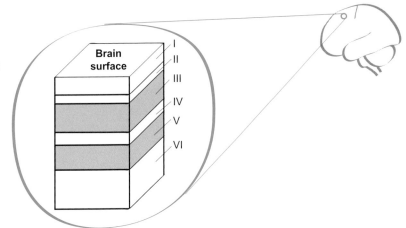

Broca's area (8A) controls **speech motor** function and is **lateralized**, i.e. present on only one side of the brain. In about 80 per cent of people it is present in the **left hemisphere**. The **auditory cortex (8B)** processes **acoustic information**. It receives contralateral information via the ipsilateral **medial geniculate nucleus** (MGN). Spatial representation occurs in the auditory area with respect to pitch of sounds. The **pons (8C)** is divided into **basal** (longitudinal fibre bundles and transverse fibres) and **dorsal** (medullary tracts) regions. It receives **inferior, middle** and **superior cerebellar peduncles** and contains the **medial lemniscus** and **pontine nucleus** which give off ponto-cerebellar fibres. The **motor cortex (8D)** receives afferent fibres from the **thalamus** and **motor fibres** which end up in the lateral and ventral **corticospinal tracts** originate here.

Answers
6. F F F F T
7. T T T T F
8. See explanation

9. Look at the cross section of the brain below and label the structures indicated

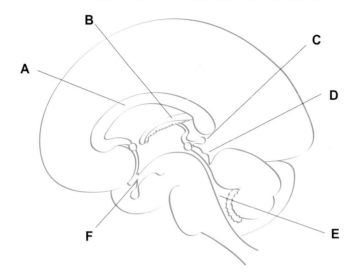

10. Look at the cross section of the brain below and label the structures indicated

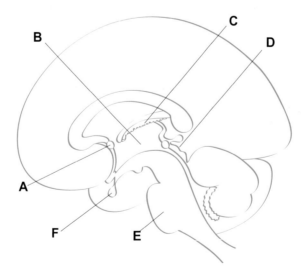

ACTH, adenocorticotrophic hormone; ADH, antidiuretic hormone; CSF, cerebrospinal fluid; FSH, follicle stimulating hormone; LH, luteinising hormone; TSH, thyroid stimulating hormone

EXPLANATION: NEUROANATOMY (i)

9A. **Corpus callosum**. This tract acts as a **bridge** where 300 million fibres cross over between the two hemispheres. In severe poorly controlled epilepsy, the corpus callosum may be cut to prevent seizures spreading from one hemisphere to another.

9B. **Fornix.** The fornix is a **bilateral bundle of fibres** that connects the **hippocampus** (located in the temporal lobe) with the **hypothalamus**. It is considered to be part of the **limbic system**.

9C. **Pineal gland.** This gland stores and releases **melatonin**. In humans melatonin levels drop at puberty and it appears that this helps stimulate growth of the reproductive organs. In mammals pineal activity is influenced by light – melatonin synthesis increases in darkness.

9D. **Inferior colliculus.** This is a **nucleus** in the **auditory pathway** and fibres connect it to the **medial geniculate nucleus** in the **thalamus** (the superior colliculus is part of the visual pathway and is connected to the lateral geniculate nucleus).

9E. **Fourth ventricle.** The fourth ventricle is a space filled with **CSF**. CSF flows into the fourth ventricle from the third ventricle via the **aqueduct** (sometimes called the **aqueduct of Sylvius**) and drains into the **subarachnoid space** through the **foramen of Magendie** and **foramen of Luschka**.

9F. **Infundibulum.** This is the mediobasal part of the hypothalamus and contains the pituitary stalk.

10A. **Anterior commissure.** The anterior commissure is a **fibre bundle** which facilitates additional communication between the **temporal lobes**. This structure assists in bilateral memory formation.

10B. **Third ventricle.** This structure is located in the **diencephalon**. CSF enters bilaterally through the paired **interventricular foramen** and exits through the **aqueduct**.

10C. **Choroid plexus.** The choroid plexus is made up of **ependymal cells** which form an epithelium. The cells **secrete CSF** and are found in the ventricles.

10D. **Superior colliculus.** This is part of the visual system, receiving fibres from the **visual cortex**. It is involved in eye and head movements.

10E. **Pons.** See page 65.

10F. **Pituitary gland.** The pituitary gland **secretes** a variety of **hormones**. The **posterior** part of the gland has a **nerve supply** and secretes **oxytocin** and **vasopressin** (**ADH**)). The **anterior** part of the pituitary secretes **FSH**, **LH**, **growth hormone**, **TSH**, **prolactin** and **ACTH**.

Answers
9. See explanation
10. See explanation

11. **Look at the cross section of the brain below and label the structures indicated**

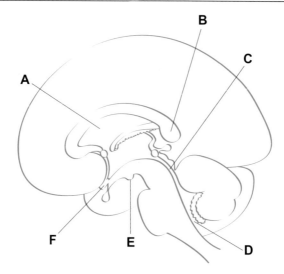

12. **In the cerebral cortex**

    a. The primary auditory area is located on the middle temporal gyrus
    b. There is a sensory homunculus in both parietal lobes
    c. Visual cortex lies inferiorly and superiorly to the calcarine sulcus
    d. The secondary olfactory area is located in the uncus
    e. The speech motor area is located in the left inferior frontal gyrus

EXPLANATION: NEUROANATOMY (ii)

11A. **Septum pellucidum**. A thin sheet of **neuroglial tissue** which bridges the gap between the corpus callosum and the fornix.

11B. **Splenium**. This is the **posterior** part of the **corpus callosum**.

11C. **Cerebral aqueduct**. The aqueduct permits **CSF** to **flow** from the **third** to the **fourth ventricles**.

11D. **Median aperture of Magendie**. The median aperture of Magendie is an opening which allows **CSF** to flow out through the **fourth ventricle** into the **subarachnoid space**.

11E. **Mammillary body**. These distinctive structures send fibres to the **thalamus** and receive fibres from the **fornix**. In Korsakov's syndrome they may show haemorrhagic damage – this can be detected on MRI.

11F. **Optic chiasm**. The optic chiasm is a crossroads for **optic fibres** from the **retina**. It is an important x-shaped structure. This is discussed in more detail on page 85.

Answers
11. See explanation
12. F T T F T

13. Select the correct labels for the figure from the list below

Options

A. Oculomotor nerve
B. Nerve which carries acoustic and positional information
C. Posterior cerebral artery
D. Blood vessel which arises directly from the internal carotid artery
E. Blood vessel which arises from the posterior communicating artery
F. A lesion here would cause contralateral paralysis below the neck
G. A lesion here would cause ipsilateral paralysis below the neck
H. An ascending sensory tract
I. Vagus nerve
J. Hypoglossal nerve

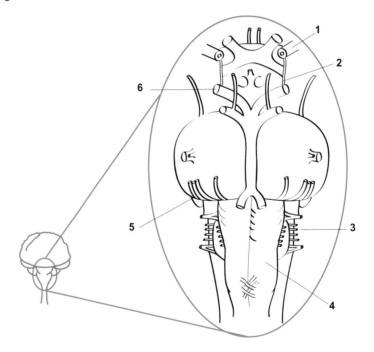

EXPLANATION: THE BRAINSTEM

The **brainstem** consists of the **medulla, pons** and **midbrain**. It is connected to the cerebellum by **three cerebellar peduncles**. The brainstem contains the nuclei for **cranial nerves III to XII** and also contains centres which help govern control of **breathing, consciousness** (arousal), **eye movements** and the **cardiovascular system**.

The **arterial blood supply** for the cerebral hemispheres is derived from the two **internal carotid arteries** and two **vertebral arteries**. These anastomose to form the **arterial circle of Willis**. The circular structure of the arterial circle means the cerebral vessels are still perfused even if a blockage in one of the small intercommunicating arteries occurs.

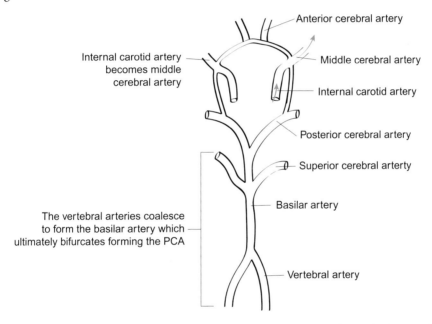

A lesion at 4 would cause contralateral paralysis since the motor neuron fibres that are cut here have not yet decussated.

13. 1 – D, 2 – A, 3 – I, 4 – F, 5 – B1, 6 – C

14. Label the structures in the horizontal section of the brain, using the options below

Options

A. Part of the lateral ventricle
B. This structure receives afferent fibres from the medial lemniscus
C. This part of the brain is involved in processing olfactory information
D. This structure is supplied by the middle meningeal artery
E. This bundle is part of a system which influences emotion

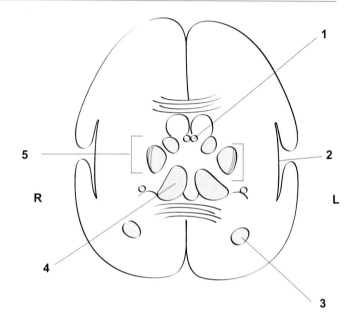

15. The medial lemniscus

a. Includes fibres from the gracile and cuneate nucleus
b. Terminates in the thalamus at the ventroposterior nucleus
c. Is ventral to the pyramid
d. Ascends through the internal capsule
e. Carries pain and temperature information

16. In the medulla

a. The superior, middle and inferior cerebellar peduncles are not intimately related
b. The olive marks the position of the inferior olivary nucleus
c. The hypoglossal nerve arises dorsal to the olive
d. The pyramids are inferior to the pons
e. The ninth, tenth and eleventh nerves are grouped together

CT, computed tomography; MRI, magnetic resonance imaging

EXPLANATION: THE MIDBRAIN

In this **horizontal** (or **transverse**) section through the brain it is conventional to look at the image **upwards** i.e. from below, up. This is how CT and MRI scans are scrutinized, so it's never too early to get used to it! This also means that left and right are reversed. The **lateral ventricles** are **bilateral** c-shaped spaces – the posterior horn of the lateral ventricles is more inferior than the anterior horn, so it is the only part shown. The position of the slice is shown below.

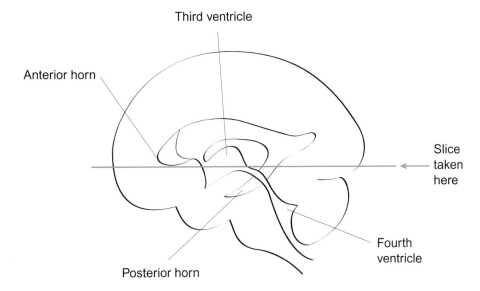

B is the thalamus, which **receives sensory afferent fibres**, including those of the **medial lemniscus**, and sends relays to the cortex. **C** is the **uncus** and is the **olfactory** centre in the brain. **D** is the **corpus striatum** and is supplied by the **middle meningeal artery** (for more on the blood supply of the brain see page 65). **E** is the **fornix**, which is part of the **limbic system** and influences **emotion**.

The **medial lemniscus** (lemniscus = ribbon) is a tract which carries **sensory information** from the **gracile** (information from the leg and lower trunk) and **cuneate** (information from the arm and the upper part of the trunk) **nuclei**. The fibres of the medial lemniscus **decussate** in the lower part of the **medulla** and travel upwards to terminate in the **ventroposterior nucleus** of the **thalamus**. The internal capsule carries descending motor and sensory fibres only, not ascending fibres.

See page 47 for a diagram of the brainstem.

---

17. The thalamus

a. Medially forms part of the third ventricular wall
b. Has a blood supply from the anterior cerebral artery
d. Is superior to the body of the fornix
d. Is separated from the lentiform nucleus by the posterior limb of the internal capsule
e. Contains numerous nuclei

18. The thalamus

a. Is part of the midbrain
c. Includes the lateral geniculate nucleus

b. Releases hormones
d. Receives fibres from the cerebellum
e. Sends motor fibres to the spinal cord

19. The cerebellum

a. Lies below the tentorium cerebelli
c. Lies within the posterior fossa
e. Receives part of its blood supply from the vertebral artery

b. Forms the roof of the rhomboid fossa
d. Is connected to the midbrain by three pairs of peduncles

20. Study the diagram of the cerebellum and answer the questions below

A. Is this an inferior or superior view of the cerebellum?
B. Which lobe is this?
C. What is the name of this structure?
D. What is the anatomical term for this structure?

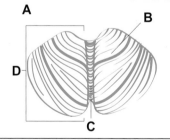

21. Consider the hindbrain

a. Pontocerebellar fibres travel through the superior cerebellar peduncles
b. It contains the basal ganglia
c. A lesion to the gracile nucleus causes ipsilateral anaesthesia
d. The glossopharyngeal nerve arises dorsal to the olive
e. It contains the respiratory centre

LGN, lateral geniculate nucleus; MGN, medial geniculate nucleus; VPL, ventral posterolateral nucleus

EXPLANATION: THE MIDBRAIN AND THE HINDBRAIN

The **thalamus** and **internal capsule** are supplied mainly by the **middle cerebral artery** and to a small extent by the **posterior cerebral artery** – the reliance on the middle cerebral artery is evident in a stroke when its occlusion may wipe out large tracts of the internal capsule causing contralateral hemiplegia – see page 67. The thalamus is part of the **diencephalon** and is an important relay centre for sensory neurons – it has very little direct motor function. It contains many nuclei – every nucleus in the thalamus (apart from the reticular nucleus) **sends fibres** to the **cortex**, and **receives sensory fibres** from all over the body including the cerebellum. The most important ones to remember are the **VPL**, the **LGN** and the **MGN**.

The cerebellum is separated superiorly from the occipital lobe by the **tentorium cerebelli** – an **infolding** of the **dural** membrane and occupies the **posterior fossa** of the **cranium**. The cerebellum forms the roof of the fourth ventricle – removal of the cerebellum exposes the diamond-shaped walls of the fourth ventricle (the **rhomboid fossa**). The cerebellum is connected to all three parts of the brainstem:

Midbrain → Superior cerebellar peduncles ↘

Pons → Middle cerebellar peduncles → Cerebellum

Medulla → Inferior cerebellar peduncles ↗

As their name suggests, the **pontocerebellar fibres** 20A originate in the pons which means they pass through the middle cerebellar peduncles. In question 20, the superior surface of the cerebellum is shown. Like the cerebrum, the cerebellum has lobes. 20B is the **anterior lobe**. The others are the **middle** and **posterior** lobes. 20C is the **vermis** and 20D is a **hemisphere**, again analogous to the cerebrum.

The **hindbrain** is composed of the **medulla**, **pons** and **cerebellum**. It is too inferior to contain any parts of the **basal ganglia** which occupy the **midbrain** and **diencephalon**. A lesion to either the **gracile** or **cuneate nucleus** causes an ispsilateral sensory deficit as the fibres decussate superiorly.

Answers
17. T F F T T
18. F F T T F
19. T T T F T
20. See explanation
21. F F F T T

22. Consider the cranial nerves

a. The optic nerve originates in the brainstem
b. The III and IV cranial nerves only are responsible for eye movements
c. The trochlear nerve exits the brainstem ventrally
d. Bell's palsy may occur if the trigeminal nerve is compressed
e. The facial nerve has six branches to the facial muscles

23. Consider the cranial nerve nuclei

a. The nuclei are paired
b. The nucleus ambiguus is a motor nucleus of the vagus nerve
c. The spinal nucleus of the trigeminal nerve has a motor function
d. The hypoglossal nucleus has motor and sensory function
e. The trochlear nuclei supplies fibres to the ipsilateral superior oblique muscle

24. Match each of the cranial nerves labelled on the figure below with one of the following options

Options

A. Damage to this nerve may cause Bell's palsy
B. Provides motor innervation to the tongue
C. Damage to this nerve may cause vertigo and tinnitus
D. Elevates the soft palate
E. Provides sensory supply to the teeth
F. Supplies the trapezius

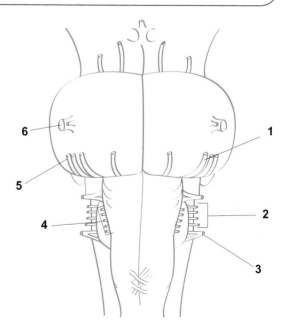

EXPLANATION: THE CRANIAL NERVES

The **optic nerve** does not originate in the brainstem, its axons arise from **ganglion cells** in the retina. The **extraocular muscles** of the eye (the muscles that move the eyeball) are supplied by cranial nerves **III**, **IV** and **VI**. For a more detailed explanation of this mechanism, see page 85. Damage to cranial nerve **VIII** (facial) may cause **Bell's palsy** – ispilateral weakness of the facial muscles. The **facial nerve** is mostly motor in function and has five branches to the facial muscles. An easy way of remembering them is the acronym – '**two zombies buggered my cat**' (temporal, zygomatic, buccal, mandibular, cervical). The facial nerve supplies the taste component of the two-thirds of the tongue via the **chorda tympani nerve**.

The **trigeminal nerve** has both **motor** and **sensory** roles and has separate pairs of motor and sensory nuclei. The trigeminal nerve has three branches – the **opthalmic, maxillary** and **mandibular branches**. It also supplies the **muscles of mastication** (those used for eating).

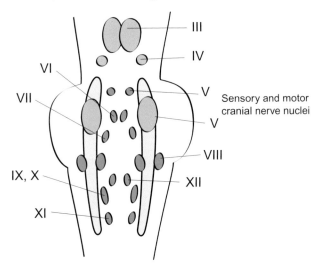

Cranial nerve **X (vagus)** has three pairs of cranial nuclei – the **nucleus ambiguus** (motor), the **dorsal nucleus** (secretomotor parasympathetic – it causes glands such as the mucous, gastric and salivary glands to secrete) and the **solitary nucleus** (sensory – think solitary = sensory). The spinal **trigeminal nucleus** receives pain information. The **hypoglossal nerve** innervates the muscles of the tongue – it has no sensory function. The trochlear nerve supplies the **contralateral superior oblique muscle** of the eye. This is the only cranial nerve that exits from the **dorsal surface** of the brainstem and **decussates**.

25. The spinal cord

a. Contains the neuronal circuitry for the monosynaptic reflex arc   7
b. Is thicker in the cervical and lumbosacral areas   7
c. Has 32 pairs of spinal nerves   F
d. Contains nerve cell bodies in the white matter   F
e. Is enveloped by three membranes   F

26. Cervical dorsal root fibres

a. Include sensory fibres
b. Are fewer in number than ventral root fibres
c. Include nerve fibres that synapse with the cuneate nucleus
d. Include non-myelinated axons
e. Contain pseudobipolar neurons

27. On the spinal cord cross section below identify the structures shown and briefly describe their role in the CNS

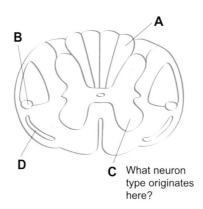

A
B
D
C   What neuron type originates here?

CNS, central nervous system

EXPLANATION: THE SPINAL CORD

The **spinal cord thickens** in the **cervical** and **lumbosacral** regions because of the presence of **increased sensory** and **motor neuronal supply** to the arms and legs. The spinal cord has **31 pairs** of spinal nerves – the vertebral column has 32 vertebrae. The dark matter is made up of cell bodies – white matter is light in colour because it is composed of myelinated nerve fibre tracts which contain lots of lipids, not cell bodies. The spinal cord is bounded with **three membranes** as is the rest of the CNS – the **pia mater** (innermost), **arachnoid membrane** and the outermost membrane, the **dura mater**.

The **gracile fasciculus (27A)** carries **sensory information** to the **somatosensory cortex** from the lower limbs. The **left rubrospinal tract (27B)** has a motor function, thought to have a role in the control of flexor and extensor muscles. These fibres arise in the red nucleus.

There are two types of neuron that originate at 27C: **alpha-motor neurons** – large diameter motor neurons which **supply** the **extrafusal fibres** of **skeletal muscles**; these are second order neurons and receive their input from the first order neurons which arise from the motor cortex of the brain. **gamma-motor neurons** also arise here – these are smaller diameter motor neurons which **supply** the **intrafusal fibres** of **muscle spindles**.

The **spinothalamic tract (27D)** carries **pain** and **temperature information.** This tract arises from second order sensory neurons which project from laminae I, III, IV of the posterior grey horn.

Answers
25. T T F F F
26. T F T F T
27. See explanation

28. On the spinal cord cross section below identify the structures shown and briefly describe their role in the CNS

    A. What is this tract? State the effect of a lesion on it in the spinal cord.
    B. The cell bodies for which neurons lie here?
    C. Where in the brain do these fibres originate?
    D. What is this structure? List four sensory modalities transmitted through it.

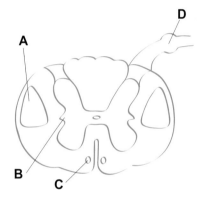

29. What changes would you expect to see upon examination on the right side of a man with a right-sided hemisection of the spinal cord at level T4?

    A. Reduced pain and temperature sensation in his arm
    B. Hyperreflexia in the knee and ankle
    C. Extensor plantar response
    D. Loss of proprioception in the great toe
    E. Loss of sensation around the right nipple

30. The following would suggest an upper motor neuron lesion

    a. Muscle wasting   **b.** Loss of muscle tone
    c. Hypereflexia   **d.** Fasciculation
    e. Extensor plantar response

CNS, central nervous system

EXPLANATION: THE SPINAL CORD

The **left lateral corticospinal tract** (28A) is the major **voluntary motor pathway**; **85 per cent** of the corticospinal tract **decussates** at the **pyramids.** Injury to these fibres below this level results in **paralysis** on the same side as the spinal cord lesion. **Sixty to eighty per cent** of its fibres originate in the **primary motor cortex.** Other fibres arise from the **supplementary motor cortex, premotor cortex** and the **somatosensory cortex.**

Cell bodies of **pre-ganglionic sympathetic motor neurones** (28B) are only found in the thoracic region of the spinal cord.

The fibres of the **ventral corticospinal tract** (28C) arise from the **primary motor cortex, premotor cortex** and **somatosensory cortex** with those that form the lateral corticospinal tract. The bulk of descending motor fibres decussate at the pyramids (85 per cent), the remaining 15 per cent continue downward without crossing over (until near their terminals) to form the ventral corticospinal tract.

The sensory modalities of the **dorsal root ganglion (posterior root ganglion)**(28D) are **pain, temperature, proprioception, crude touch, fine touch** and **vibration**.

Answers
28. See explanation
29. F T T T T
30. F F T T T

31. The peripheral nervous system

a. Includes the spinal cord
b. Is made up of the spinal cord and spinal nerve
c. Is found outside the spinal cord
d. Includes the sympathetic chain
e. Is made up of efferent nerve fibres

32. Complete the numbered statements below from the options given

Options

A. Axons
B. Cell bodies
C. A-delta fibres
D. Dendrites
E. Dorsal root
F. C fibres
G. Motor neurons
H. Ventral horn
I. Dorsal horn
J. Substantia gelatinosa

1. Ganglia are a collection of ......
2. A nerve is a collection of ......
3. Sensory ganglia are found in the ......
4. Motor ganglia are found in the ......
5. The largest diameter nerve fibres are ......

33. Label the figure opposite using the options below

Options

A. Spinal nerve
B. Sympathetic ganglion
C. Motor neuron
D. White matter
E. Interneuron
F. Small intestine
G. Pacinian corpuscle
H. Pre-ganglionic autonomic neuron
I. Sensory neuron
J. Dorsal root ganglion
K. Skeletal muscle
L. Grey matter
M. Dorsal root
N. Ventral root
O. Blood vessel

ANS, autonomic nervous system; CNS, central nervous system; PNS, peripheral nervous system

EXPLANATION: PERIPHERAL NERVOUS SYSTEM

The nervous system is divided into **three** main divisions – the **CNS** the **PNS** and the **ANS**.

- The CNS is made up of the brain and spinal cord and includes the eye
- The PNS is defined as those nerves which lie outside the brain and spinal cord
- The ANS has components in both the CNS and PNS, and has a special regulatory role throughout the body

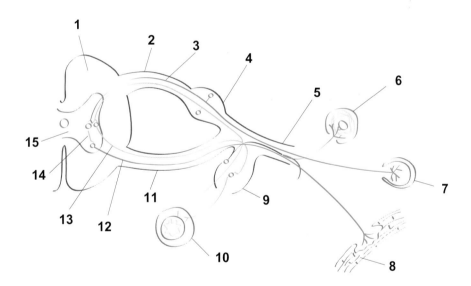

Answers
31. F F T T F
32. 1– B, 2 – A, 3 – E, 4 – H, 5 – E
33. 1 – D, 2 – M, 3 – I, 4 – J, 5 – A, 6 – O, 7 – G, 8 – K, 9 – B, 10 – F, 11 – N, 12 – C, 13, – H, 14 – E, 15 – L

34. Complete the diagram below of the target organs and the innervating structures themselves of the autonomic nervous system

Options

A. Lung

B. Adrenal gland

C. Vagus nerve

D. Eye

E. Large intestine and rectum

F. Bladder and reproductive organs

G. Tear and salivary glands

H. Inferior mesenteric ganglion

I. Coeliac ganglion

J. Superior cervical ganglion

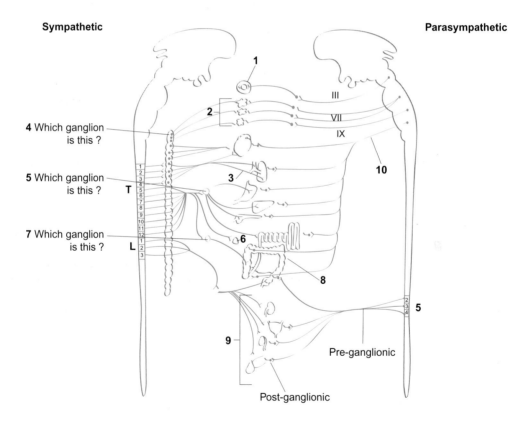

Sympathetic

Parasympathetic

1

2

III

VII

IX

4 Which ganglion is this ?

5 Which ganglion is this ?

T

3

10

7 Which ganglion is this ?

L

6

8

5

9

Pre-ganglionic

Post-ganglionic

EXPLANATION: THE AUTONOMIC NERVOUS SYSTEM

The functions of the **viscera** (the organs of the abdomen and thorax i.e. kidney, intestines and heart) and other **innervated smooth muscle** (e.g. the intraocular muscles) and secretory cells (the islets of Langerhan's) are controlled by the **ANS**. The ANS has three branches: **sympathetic**, **parasympathetic** and **enteric**. The **sympathetic** branch of the ANS takes over during periods of **stress**, dilating the bronchi of the lungs, reducing gastric motility, constricting blood vessels to increase blood pressure, increasing heart rate and contractility, while input from the parasympathetic nervous system is reduced. At rest the parasympathetic branch has a greater input. The actions of the ANS are summarized in the table below.

Organ	Sympathetic	Parasympathetic
Eye	Pupillary dilation	Pupillary constriction
Lacrimal and salivary glands	Inhibition of secretion	Increase in secretion
Lungs	Bronchodilation Inhibition of secretion	Bronchoconstriction Increase in secretion
Heart	Increase in heart rate Increase in contractility	Reduction of heart rate
Adrenal gland	Release of medullary hormones	No innervation
Stomach and small intestine	Inhibition of peristalsis and secretions	Increase in peristalsis and secretions
Large intestine	Inhibition of peristalsis and secretions	Increased smooth muscle tone
Reproductive organs	Ejaculation	Erection

Remember '**point** and **shoot**' (**parasympathetic = erection, sympathetic = ejaculation**). Both branches have **pre-** and **post-ganglionic** fibres, the only exception is the sympathetic nerve supply to the **adrenal medulla** which does not. The **sympathetic** supply is derived from the **thoracic** and **lumbar** parts of the spinal cord, the **parasympathetic** supply comes **from cranial nerves III, VII, IX and X** and the **sacral** part of the spinal cord.

The enteric part of the ANS is confined to the gut lining and receives efferents from the sympathetic and parasympathetic branches.

Answers
34. 1 – D, 2 – G, 3 – A, 4 – J, 5 – I, 6 – B, 7 – H, 8 – E, 9 – F, 10 – C

35. CSF is located

a. In the cerebral blood vessels
b. In the peripheral circulation
c. In the ventricles of the brain
d. In the central canal of the spinal cord
e. In the anterior chamber of the eye

36. Consider the ventricular system of the brain

a. The lateral ventricles are inferior to the hypothalamus
b. The choroid plexus is found in the third ventricle
c. Cerebrospinal fluid (CSF) is only secreted in the anterior horns of the lateral ventricles
d. The thalamus forms part of the floor of the fourth ventricle
e. The lateral ventricles drain into the third ventricle via the foramen of Lushka

37. Examine the diagram of the brain below

A. Indicate on the diagram one site where CSF is made
B. What is the name of this meningeal compartment?
C. Name C. What structures permit the flow of CSF through B into C?

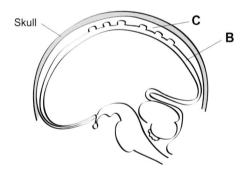

Skull

C

B

38. Cerebrospinal fluid

a. Is only formed in the third and fourth ventricles
b. Is slowly turned over
c. Passes between the lateral ventricles by the cerebral aqueduct
d. May enter the circulation through the sigmoid venous sinus
e. The total volume of CSF is between 80 and 150ml

CNS, central nervous system; CSF, cerebrospinal fluid; Cl⁻, chloride ion, K⁺, potassium ion; Na⁺, sodium ion

EXPLANATION: CEREBROSPINAL FLUID

The brain is bathed in cerebrospinal fluid (CSF). It protects and helps support the brain metabolically and mechanically.

CSF is a **clear watery fluid** found throughout the **ventricular** system of the CNS. It is secreted from the **ependymal** cells of the **choroid plexus** in the **lateral**, **third** and **fourth ventricles**.

CSF is formed mostly in the lateral ventricles and to a lesser extent in the third and fourth ventricles (37A). It is turned over relatively quickly at a rate of about 500 ml/day. The lateral ventricles are connected by the **interventricular foramen** – the cerebral **aqueduct** connects the third and fourth ventricles. The CSF occupies the **subarachnoid space** (37B) and passes into the **venous sinuses** (the **sagittal** (37C) and **sigmoid** sinuses) via the **arachnoid granulations**. The neural membranes and CSF circulation are shown below.

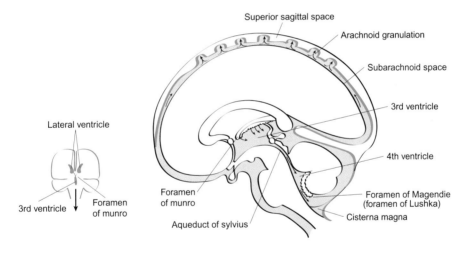

The brain's main fuel is **glucose**, levels of which are **tightly controlled** in the CNS. Under resting conditions, the brain accounts for 15 per cent of the total metabolism of the body but is only 2 per cent of the body's mass. A comparison between the major constituents of plasma and the CSF is shown below – the most significant difference is that of protein concentration.

	Plasma	CSF
Na^+ (mM)	150	150
K^+ (mM)	4	3
Cl^- (mM)	120	130
Glucose (mM)	6	4
Protein (mg/(100 g))	6500	25

Answers
35. F F T T F
36. F T F F F
37. See explanation
38. F F F T T

39. Match the structures in the numbered list to the blood vessels that supply them

Options

A. Posterior cerebral artery
C. Basilar artery
E. Middle cerebral artery

B. Superior cerebellar artery
D. Anterior cerebral artery

1. Pons
3. Auditory area
5. Visual area

2. Broca's area
4. Cerebellum

40. Which blood vessels (from the same lettered list) supply the shaded parts shown in the figures below?

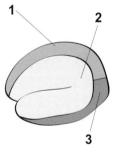

Lateral surface of the
left hemisphere

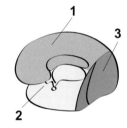

Medial surface of the
right hemisphere

41. Consider maintenance of the brain

a. Fatty acids may cross the blood–brain barrier
b. Protein levels are greater in CSF than plasma
c. Glucose is the main source of energy
d. CSF is formed from glial cells
e. CSF is found in the subarachnoid space

CSF, cerebrospinal fluid

EXPLANATION: BLOOD SUPPLY TO THE BRAIN

The **pons** is supplied by the **basilar artery**, and the **superior cerebellar artery** supplies the **cerebellum** along with several other blood vessels. **Broca's area** and the **auditory area** are both supplied by the **middle cerebral artery**. The **visual area** is supplied by the **posterior cerebral artery**. The blood supply to these areas can be seen in the figure below.

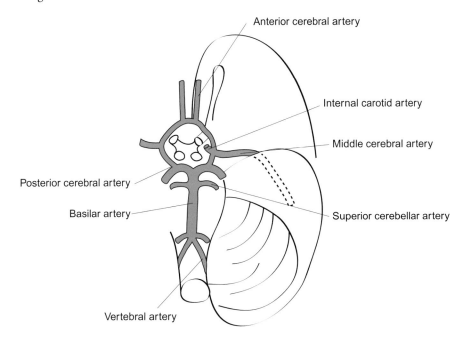

Anterior cerebral artery

Internal carotid artery

Middle cerebral artery

Posterior cerebral artery

Basilar artery

Superior cerebellar artery

Vertebral artery

Fatty acids cannot cross the **blood–brain barrier**; however, in times of glucose deficiency (starvation) the body gets around this by **converting fatty acids** to **ketone bodies** which can cross over into the brain.

42. Concerning stroke diagnosis

Mr Johnson is a 56 year-old Afro-Caribbean man who is brought into the emergency department one evening. He works as a cabinet maker and was planing some oak panelling when he suddenly lost consciousness and collapsed. He was found shortly afterwards by his daughter. On regaining consciousness he is alert but his speech is slurred and neurological examination shows profound weakness and sensory loss in the right side of his body. Mr Johnson has been a diabetic for eight years and smokes 20 cigarettes a day.

    A. What is the likely diagnosis?

    B. Explain in anatomical terms what has happened.

    C. Are there any factors in the history which may have predisposed Mr Johnson to this condition? Suggest two others.

    D. What is the likelihood of the same condition affecting Mr Johnson's children in the future?

CVA, cerebrovascular accident; MRI, magnetic resonance imaging

EXPLANATION: STROKE

Mr Johnson has had a **stroke**, or CVA (A). Since the deficit is on the **right side** of his body, it is highly likely that the occluded artery is in the **left side** of the brain, because the **corticospinal** (motor) and the **gracile** and **cuneate** (sensory) pathways both **decussate** in the medulla (B).

The fact that such a large part of his body is affected by the stroke means that the **blood supply** to both **somatosensory** and **motor** areas of the **cortex** has been **compromised**. The cortex in this area is supplied by the **middle cerebral artery** – therefore its occlusion probably accounts for his condition.

Some important predisposing factors to stroke are (C):

• Smoking – damages vascular endothelium and causes atherosclorosis
• Hypertension – increased risk of dislodged thrombus
• Atrial fibrillation – risk of thrombus formation in the atria of the heart
• Diabetes – damages vascular endothelium and causes atherosclerosis
• Ethnic origin – Afro-Caribbean and Indian individuals have greater stroke incidence

There is a **strong hereditary component** to **diabetes** and the **ethnic** origin of the children puts them at risk of **developing hypertension** and **stroke**. **Smoking** is a modifiable risk factor and may or may not apply to this man's children. Overall there is a **moderate** to **strong** chance that Mr Johnson's children will suffer a CVA at some stage in their lives (D).

Answers
42. See explanation

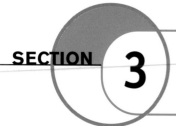

SECTION 3

SENSORY SYSTEMS

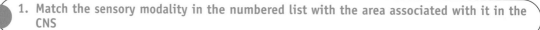

1. Match the sensory modality in the numbered list with the area associated with it in the CNS

Options

A. Striate cortex
B. Pyriform cortex
C. Inferior colliculus
D. Periaqueductal grey matter
E. Somatosensory cortex

1. Olfaction
2. Gustation
3. Vision
4. Touch
5. Hearing

2. Olfactory epithelial cells

a. Line most of the nasal cavity
b. Are ciliated
c. May be pigmented
d. Cover five times the surface area in the domestic cat
e. Degenerate and are replaced after approximately one year

3. Consider olfaction

a. It is mediated by cyclic adenosine monophosphate (cAMP)
b. It is not well understood
c. Two chemically dissimilar substances may produce similar smells
d. Optical isomers frequently have similar smells
e. It is an important component of taste

cAMP, cyclic adenosine monophosphate; CNS, central nervous system

EXPLANATION: SENSATION AND OLFACTION

Olfactory epithelial cells are responsible for **scent detection**. In humans the olfactory epithelium lines only a **small portion** of the **nasal cavity**. The epithelium is made up of olfactory (smell) receptor cells which each have around 8–20 cilia. The olfactory epithelial cells have a high turnover rate and are replaced every month. These receptor cells send axons up through the **cribiform plate** to synapse in the **olfactory bulb**. The nasal cavity is shown in a parasagittal section of the human head below.

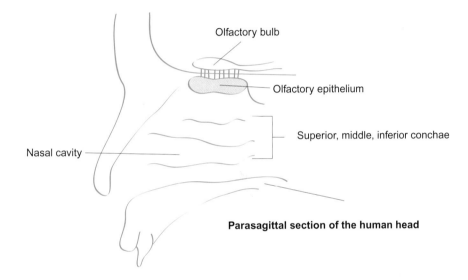

Parasagittal section of the human head

The physiology of olfaction is poorly understood. It is known that the cell membrane's response to a scent stimulus is relatively long i.e. it is depolarized for seconds, not milliseconds and that it is modulated by cAMP. The chemical structure of odorants (scent molecules) has little bearing on the type of olfactory sensation they produce. Camphor and hexachloroethane for example are very different molecules structurally and chemically but both smell similar. Scent is an important component of taste – a blocked nose will significantly alter taste sensation.

Answers
1. 1 – B, 2 – B, 3 – A, 4 – E, 5 – C
2. F T T T F
3. T T T T T

4. Olfaction and gustation

a. Anosmia refers to loss of taste sensation
b. There are five gustatory modalities
c. Scent receptors in a dog are more sensitive than in man
d. Gustatory receptors respond best to short stimuli
e. Olfaction and gustation are both functions of the motor system

5. Choose the option from the list below that best matches each of the numbered points

Options

A. Cranial nerve VII
B. Cranial nerve IX
C. Cranial nerve V
D. Cranial nerve X
E. Towards
F. Away
G. No change

1. Somatic sensation is supplied by ......
2. Taste in the anterior two-thirds of the tongue is supplied by ......
3. Taste in the posterior one-third of the tongue is supplied by ......
4. The chorda tympani is a branch of which nerve?
5. Damage to the motor supply to one side of the tongue causes it to move in which direction in relation to the lesion?

EXPLANATION: OLFACTION AND GUSTATION

The **nerve supply** to the **tongue** is quite varied, but it is worth knowing as examiners seem to love it.

The **motor** supply to the tongue is from cranial nerve **XII (hypoglossal nerve)**.

General **sensation** (touch, pain, temperature) is served by cranial nerve **V (trigeminal nerve)**.

Taste in the **anterior two-thirds** of the tongue is supplied by cranial nerve **VII (facial nerve)**; in the **posterior one-third** of the tongue it is supplied by cranial nerve **IX (glossopharyngeal nerve)**.

If the motor supply to the tongue is damaged, on sticking out the tongue, it will deviate towards the side of the lesion (due to the muscles being weaker on that side).

Answers
4. F T F T F
5. 1 – C, 2 – A, 3 – B, 4 – A, 5 – E

6. Consider events in light receptor cells

a. Light energy causes conjugation of opsin and retinal
b. All-*trans* retinal is converted to 11-*cis* retinal by an isomerase enzyme
c. In darkness most rhodopsin is in its bleached form
d. Reconversion of 11-*cis* retinal to all-trans retinal is a relatively slow process
e. Reconversion of 11-*cis* retinal to all-*trans* retinal is slower in cones than rods

7. Label the illustration of the rhodopsin-retinal visual cycle using the options below.

Options

A. 11-*cis* retinal
B. All-trans-retinol (vitamin A)
C. Rhodopsin
D. 11-*cis* retinol
E. Free opsin

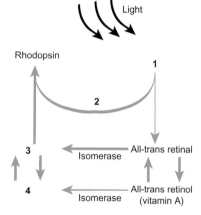

8. Complete the statements in the numbered list using the options below

Options

A. cGMP
B. cAMP
C. Na+ and Ca2+
D. Na+ and cGMP
E. Na+ and cAMP
F. Increased
G. Decreased
H. Not affected

Following light stimulus in the light receptor cell
1. Activity of phosphodiesterase is ......
2. There is a decrease in the second messenger known as ......
3. Activation of ion channels causes a decrease of intracellular ......
4. The cell membrane polarity is ......
5. Neurotransmitter release is ......

Ca2+, calcium ion; cGMP, cyclic guanosine monophosphate; Na+, sodium ion

EXPLANATION: BIOCHEMISTRY OF VISION

Light hitting the **cones** or **rods** splits the **rhodopsin** into **opsin** and **all-*trans* retinal**. In light conditions most of the rhodopsin is described as being bleached (what is meant is that it is split into opsin and retinal). Once all-*trans* retinal is formed, its conversion back to its isomer form **11-*cis* retinal** is slow compared to events in the rest of the rhodopsin cycle. This delay accounts for the slowness of rods to adapt from light to dark conditions. The **reconversion** appears to be **faster in cones than rods** as the former are specialized for bright light and have a high all-trans retinal turnover.

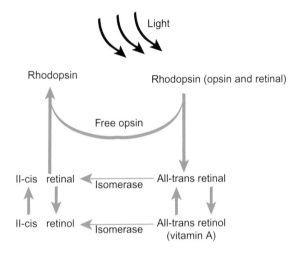

The exact mechanism of **signal transduction** in the light receptors is unclear but the following is the sequence of events:

1. Bleached rhodopsin couples with G-protein
2. This activates phosphodiesterase
3. In turn this converts cGMP to GMP
4. Decrease of cGMP causes a reduction in sodium channel activation
5. Na^+ and Ca^{2+} entry into the cell decreases
6. The cell membrane becomes hyperpolarized
7. Neurotransmitter release decreases.

So **light stimulus** causes a **decrease in firing** from cones and rods – an unusual phenomenon.

Answers
6. F T T T F
7. 1 – C, 2 – E, 3 – A, 4 – D, 5 – B
8. 1 – F, 2 – A, 3 – C, 4 – F, 5 – G

9. Consider the retina cell below and choose the correct labels for the figure

Options

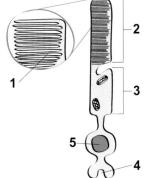

A. Rod
B. Cone
C. Amacrine cell
D. Inner segment
E. Photopigment
F. Nucleus
G. Outer segment
H. Disc
I. Synaptic terminal

6. What biochemical component here is essential for retinal signal transduction
7. What cell type is this (choose from the options above)?

10. Concerning vision

a. The human eye can detect light between 400 and 700 nm wavelength
b. Ultraviolet radiation can be seen with the naked eye
c. Dark adaptation may take up to 10 minutes
d. There are two main light receptor types in the retina
e. Cones are important for night vision

11. Cones

a. Are highly sensitive to bright light
b. Are highly concentrated in the fovea
c. Are optimally sensitive to light at a wavelength of 400 nm
d. Permit trichromatic colour discrimination
e. Play a role in high acuity vision

12. Rods

a. Are not strongly sensitive to bright light
b. Are good at detecting monochrome images
c. Adapt to brightness changes quickly
d. Are optimally sensitive to light at a wavelength of 500 nm
e. Are found in dense concentrations in the fovea

EXPLANATION: RODS AND CONES

The human eye can pick up light in the visible spectrum only – ultraviolet light lies outside this range. The retina works throughout a range of different levels of brightness – the process the eye uses to **adjust** to **different levels of brightness** is known as **adaptation**. Dark adaptation usually takes 40 minutes in a healthy subject who enters a dark room from daylight. The two main light receptor types in the retina are cones and rods. **Cones** respond best to **bright light** (think ice cream cone – daytime) and **rods** are much more sensitive and respond better to **low levels of light** (they are overloaded by bright light).

Rods and **cones** are the **light receptors** in the eye. They are composed of an inner and outer segment. The outer segment consists of a multi-invaginated plasma membrane which is folded to form **discs** or **saccules**. The membranes of these discs are covered with light-reactive **photopigments** and these are responsible for **converting light energy** into the signal which is transmitted to the visual cortex through the visual pathway. The inner segment contains the normal cellular organelles responsible for maintenance of the cell. As their name suggests, rod cells are 'rod-shaped' and cone cells are 'cone-shaped'.

Comparison of rods and cones

Cones	Rods
Low sensitivity to bright light	High sensitivity to bright light
Found in high density in the fovea	Found in low density in the fovea
Optimum light wavelength is 550 nm	Optimum light wavelength is 500 nm
Detect colour	Detect monochrome
High acuity vision	Low acuity vision
Adaptation is fast	Adaptation is slow

13. Consider the retina and select the best answer to complete the numbered questions below

The options may be used once, more than once or not at all.

Options

A. Fovea centralis   B. Amacrine cells
C. Macula lutea   D. Bipolar cells
E. The choroid   F. Horizontal cells

1. ...... is the vascular layer which supplies the cells of the retina with oxygen and nutrients
2. ...... forms a small depression in the retina
3. ...... show spike discharges in response to retinal stimulation
4. ...... is a yellow spot in the retina
5. ...... contains many more cones than rods

14. The fovea

a. Forms a blind spot
b. Is a small structure packed with rods
c. Covers approximately half the retina
d. Has the highest density of cones in the retina
e. Is colour blind because it contains no cones

15. The retina and optic nerve are all considered to be components of the

a. Peripheral nervous system   b. Auditory nervous system
c. Autonomic nervous system   d. Central nervous system
e. Gustatory nervous system

16. The retina of a wholly nocturnal animal is more likely to display which characteristic?

a. More rods than cones   b. A larger fovea than a 'day animal'
c. Poor night vision   d. Good colour vision
e. None of the above

EXPLANATION: THE RETINA

The cells of the retina are supplied by blood vessels in the **choroid layer** which lies beneath the photorecep-
tors and is separated from them by the pigment epithelium. The **macula lutea** is a yellow spot visible in the
retina temporal to the **optic disc** (blind spot) and contains the **fovea centralis** (or fovea) which is a small
depression in the centre of the macula with a particularly high concentration of cone cells. Amacrine and ganglion cells in the retina show spike discharges in response to retinal stimulation; however, other retinal cell
types such as bipolar, rod, cone and horizontal cells, do not. This is thought to be due to their small size.

The **choroid** and the **central artery** provide the vascular supply of the retina. The penetration of the retina by
the central artery and the head of the optic nerve forms the **blind spot**. The outermost parts of the retina from
the pigmented layer to the inner nuclear layer lack capillaries. The retina is drained by the retinal veins which
feed the central vein of the retina. The **fovea** is a small depression in the retina which contains a very high proportion of **cones**. The cone cells here are of very high density, in fact a much greater density than in any other
part of the retina. This high concentration of cones provides the retina with its greatest area of **visual acuity**,
but this high acuity is only useful in daylight, since cones function poorly in low light levels.

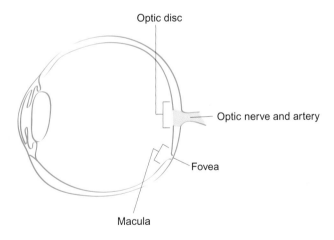

Answers
13. 1 – E, 2 – A, 3 – D, 4 – C, 5 – A
14. F F F T F
15. F F F T F
16. T F F F F

17. Label the diagram of the eye using the options given

Options

A. Conjunctiva
B. Vitreous humour
C. Iris
D. Ciliary muscle
E. Suspensory ligaments
F. Lens
G. Retina
H. Sclera
I. Aqueous humour

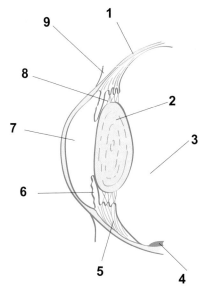

18. Consider the anterior chamber of the eye and complete the numbered statements from the options below

Options

A. The lens
B. The ciliary muscle
C. The suspensory ligaments
D. The canal of Schlemm
E. Aqueous humour

1. Fluid passes from the anterior chamber of the eye to the veins through ......
2. ...... permits accommodation in the eye through a change in shape
3. ...... are connective tissue structures around the lens
4. ...... is a plasma-like fluid containing 1 per cent of the protein found in normal plasma
5. ...... is innervated by parasympathetic fibres

EXPLANATION: THE EYE

The lens changes shape as a result of relaxation and contraction of the **ciliary muscle** (these act to thicken or flatten the lens respectively). The ciliary muscle is under **parasympathetic** control and has both **circular** and **radial** (longitudinal) muscle fibres. The **suspensory ligaments** connect the lens to the ciliary muscle. The **canal of Schlemm** permits passage of the aqueous humour produced in the anterior chamber out to the vascular system. The **aqueous humour** is produced in the ciliary body. It is similar in composition to plasma but contains 1 per cent of the protein found in plasma – its main function is to supply the lens with oxygen and nutrients.

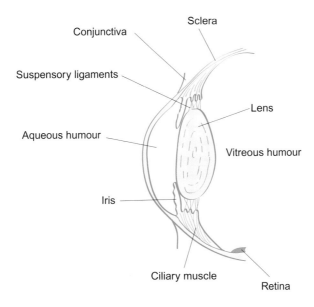

19. Consider the muscles in the eye (intraocular muscles)

Choose the effect of each of the items in the numbered list from the options given. The options may be used once, more than once or not at all

Options

A. Constriction of the lens
B. Dilatation of the lens
C. Pupillary dilation
D. Pupillary constriction
E. None of the above

1. Sphincter pupillae
2. Noradrenaline
3. Dilator pupillae
4. Atropine
5. Tropicamide

20. In the visual system

a. The image is inverted by the time it hits the retina
b. Axons from the temporal half of the retina cross in the optic chiasm
c. Signals from each half of the visual field are sent contralaterally
d. The lateral geniculate nucleus (LGN) is part of the thalamus
e. Axons of the optic radiation end in the LGN

21. Match the most specific anatomical site from the numbered list to the source of the modality in the visual pathway from the options given

Options

A. Right upper visual cortex
B. Right lower visual cortex
C. Left upper visual cortex
D. Left lower visual cortex
E. Right visual cortex
F. Left visual cortex
G. Both cortices
H. Left occipital pole
I. Right occipital pole

1. Left visual field
2. Lower right visual field
3. Right lateral geniculate nucleus
4. Left optic nerve
5. Fovea in the left retina

ACh, acetylcholine; ANS, autonomic nervous system; LGN, lateral geniculate nucleus

EXPLANATION: FUNCTIONS OF THE INTRAOCULAR MUSCLES

Accommodation, or the ability of the eye to **focus** on a fixed point, is brought about by **contraction** or **relaxation** of the ciliary muscle – this involves changes in the thickness of the lens only.

Pupil diameter is controlled by a pair of muscles – as opposed to the single muscle which is responsible for shortening and lengthening of the lens. The **sphincter pupillae** has circular muscle fibres which, when contracted, make the pupil smaller. The **dilator pupillae** has radial muscle fibres which, when contracted, cause the pupil to enlarge.

The control of pupil size is under the influence of the ANS: the parasympathetic system causes constriction, the sympathetic system causes dilation (think – wide-eyed with fright). This is illustrated alongside.

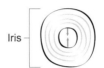

Iris

Sphincter puapillae muscles contract and constrict the iris

Dilator puapillae constricts and relaxes the iris

Sympathomimetic drugs such as **noradrenaline** cause the pupil to dilate and drugs which **antagonize** the action of **ACh** (such as **atropine**) also cause the pupil to **dilate**. **Tropicamide** is a **shorter acting muscarinic antagonist** than atropine making it more suitable for dilation of the pupil in a clinical setting and is useful for eye examinations. A large pupillary diameter is useful as it allows more light into the eye and reduces the effects of diffraction which occurs in smaller apertures. A small pupil on the other hand provides an improved depth of field and reduces inherent errors in the eye (such as an astigmatism) – looking through a pinhole can dramatically improve the vision of someone with poor eyesight.

EXPLANATION: THE VISUAL SYSTEM

Some afferent optic fibres bypass the **LGN** and terminate at other sites such as the **tegmentum**, but this is not normally considered to be core knowledge.

See overleaf for a diagram that will explain the anatomy of the visual system. Fibres from **both retinae** synapse with **both LGNs**. Fibres from the retinae do not synapse directly with the **Edinger-Westphal nucleus** – they synapse with the occulomotor nuclei – see overleaf for a diagram of the pupillary light reflex. The **internal capsule** carries afferent and efferent **sensory** and **motor** fibres to and from the **somatosensory** and **motor cortices** – it does not relay optical sensory information as this is sent to the visual cortex.

Answers
19. 1 – D, 2 – C, 3 – C, 4 – C, 5 – C
20. T F F T F
21. 1 – E, 2 – C, 3 – E, 4 – G, 5 – I

22. In the visual system

   a. 75 per cent of optic fibres cross in the optic chiasm
   b. Crossing of fibres in the chiasm is important for binocular vision
   c. All retinal fibres terminate at the lateral geniculate nucleus (LGN)
   d. The LGN has eight layers
   e. There are two pairs of LGNs in the brain

23. Label the numbered parts of the visual pathway on the figure using the options below

Options

   A. LGN
   B. Optic tract
   C. Optic chiasm
   D. Optic nerve
   E. Optic radiation
   F. Temporal retina
   G. Nasal retina

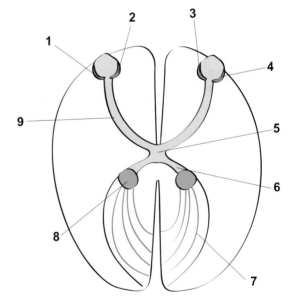

24. In the visual pathway

   a. The visual fields are represented topographically
   b. Fibres from the LGN project to the striate area
   c. The central part of the visual field is represented at the occipital pole
   d. The visual association cortex is involved in object recognition
   e. Some optic tract fibres terminate in the inferior colliculus

LGN, lateral geniculate nucleus

EXPLANATION: VISUAL PATHWAYS (i)

Information from the **visual fields** is **inverted** as it passes through the pupil and is back to front and upside down when it hits the **retina**. The retina can be divided into two functional parts – **temporal** (lateral or on the same side as the temporal bone) and **nasal** (medial or on the same side as the nasal bone). This is important because information from each half travels down a different pathway in the brain. Axons from the retina pass out through the blind spot as the optic nerve (initially following the same path as the central retinal artery); each optic nerve contains approximately one million axons.

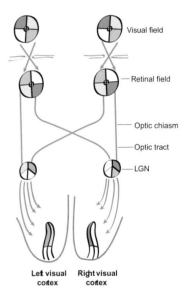

The information in the optic nerves is projected in such a way that when it reaches the visual cortex – its final destination – it is still arranged in a highly organized way. The central part of the visual field occupies a disproportionately large area of the visual cortex. This is because the **central visual field** is 'read' by the **fovea** – a part of the retina with a particularly high density of cones, which in turn send out a particularly large number of axons and thus make up a considerable part of the optic nerve. The representation of the visual fields in the visual cortex is shown opposite.

The **optic nerves** from each eye travel medially and join to form the **optic chiasm**; at this point the axons from both nasal sides of the retina cross over to the **contralateral** half of the brain and enter the **optic tract**. Axons from the **temporal** sides of the retina continue on their course in the optic tract and do not cross over. Axons from the **contralateral nasal retina** and **ipsilateral temporal retina** continue in the optic tract to the **LGN**. The LGN is a small **six-layered nucleus** in the inferior part of the **thalamus**. The crossed over nasal fibres terminate in layers 1, 4 and 6, and the ispsilateral temporal fibres terminate in layers 2, 3 and 5. Fibres leave the LGN to form the **optic radiation** which terminates in the visual cortex on both sides of the border with the **calcarine sulcus**.

25. Identify the visual deficit in each of these representations of the visual fields and mark the likely site of a lesion on the visual pathway below.

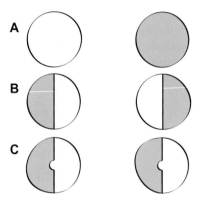

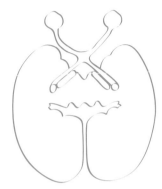

26. Study the diagram below

A. What is the name of the nucleus indicated in the diagram?
B. What two reflexes does it play a role in?
C. Briefly explain its role when light is shined into the pupil of one eye

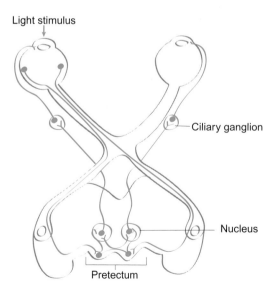

EXPLANATION: VISUAL PATHWAYS (ii)

25A. Total blindness in the right eye
25B. Bitemporal hemianopia
25C. Left homonymous hemianopia with macular sparing – this is due to ischaemic damage to the visual cortex – the macular area has a separate blood supply.

Remember, the visual fields are invertal and reversal by the time they hit the retina.

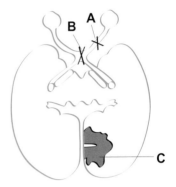

26A. Edinger-Westphal nucleus
26B. Pupillary light reflex and accommodation reflex
26C. When light hits the retina of one eye, a signal is sent through the optic nerve of that eye to the cell bodies in the pretectal area. These neurons give off ipsilateral and contralateral fibres which synapse with both Edinger-Westphal nuclei. Stimulation of both nuclei results in firing of neurons from both and results in both eyes blinking in response to a light stimulus.

The **Edinger-Westphal** nucleus is part of the **occulomotor** complex (the group of nuclei responsible for eye movements) and is located in the brainstem, posterior to the **pons**. It gives off **parasympathetic fibres** to the **ciliary ganglion** which in turn innervates the **sphincter pupillae** and **ciliary muscles** and plays a role in the two basic **occular reflexes – accommodation** and the **pupillary light reflex**. The pupillary light reflex is useful clinically as it can be evoked even in an unconscious patient and its presence is a reassuring indicator of brainstem function.

Answers
25. See explanation
26. See explanation

27. Look at the three sets of eyes below and describe the site of the lesion in each case

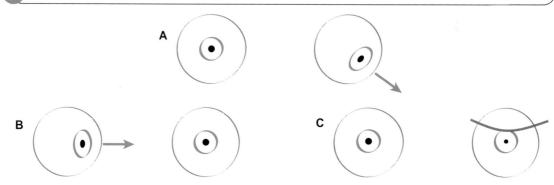

A

B

C

---

28. Problem-based question

Mrs Jones is a 72-year-old female who has smoked 20 cigarettes a day for 25 years. She is known to have a lung tumour and is seen regularly by the oncologists. She presents to the emergency department with neurological symptoms and a diagnosis of Horner's syndrome is made.

Which of the symptoms and signs below are likely to be seen in Mrs Jones?
  a. Ptosis   **b.** Large fixed pupil
  c. Small fixed pupil   **d.** Flushing and dry skin on one side of the face
  e. On protrusion the tongue deviates to one side

As a medical student in the emergency department you consider the following:
  f. Her Horner's syndrome is unlikely to be related to her tumour
  g. She is likely to have a family history of Horner's syndrome

The SHO on call examines Mrs Jones. Which of the following are possible routes of treatment?
  h. Physiotherapy   **i.** Steroids
  j. Surgery

---

29. Consider Horner's syndrome

  a. It is a common condition
  b. It is irreversible
  c. The cervical and stellate ganglia are components of the sympathetic nervous system
  d. The sympathetic chain contributes to the nerve supply of the face
  e. It is unlikely to be caused by a cerebrovascular insult

ANS, autonomic nervous system; SHO, senior house officer

EXPLANATION: HORNER'S SYNDROME

Horner's syndrome is defined as sympathetic denervation of the head i.e. damage to the superior cervical ganglion or the sympathetic chain.

Ptosis (drooping eyelid), a **small fixed pupil**, **flushing** and **warm dry skin** – usually confined to one side of the face – are all signs of **Horner's syndrome**. Anything that can disrupt the **sympathetic supply** to the head can theoretically cause Horner's syndrome e.g. trauma, stroke and degenerative disease such as multiple sclerosis. In Mrs Jones' case the tumour in her lungs has spread into the mediastinum and is **compressing** the **sympathetic chain**. Physiotherapy is unlikely to help in this case but steroid treatment may shrink the tumour enough to alleviate her symptoms. Surgery to remove the tumour may also help. Horner's syndrome is not common and may be treatable depending on the cause. Signs of Horner's syndrome are illustrated below.

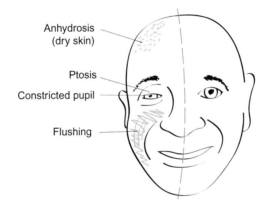

Anhydrosis (dry skin)
Ptosis
Constricted pupil
Flushing

The muscle which **elevates** the **eyelid** – the **levator palpebrae superioralis** – has dual innervation from the **sympathetic** nervous system and the **occulomotor** nerve (cranial nerve III), so ptosis is only partial if the ANS component only is damaged.

Answers
27. A – Left cranial nerve III lesion
  B – Right cranial nerve VI lesion
  C – Left-sided Horner's syndrome
28. T F T T F F F F T T
29. F F T T F

30. Consider the anatomy of the ear below and choose the correct labels from the options below

Options

A. Internal auditory meatus
B. External auditory meatus
C. Eustachian tube
D. Semicircular canal
E. Malleus
F. Stapes
G. Pinna
H. Oval window
I. Incus
J. Cochlea
K. Round window
L. Tympanic membrane
M. Cochlear nerve
N. Trigeminal nerve

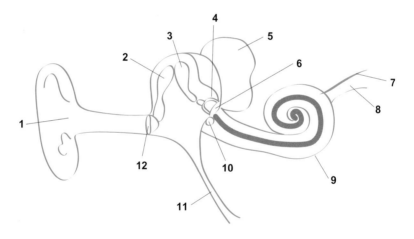

31. In the auditory system

a. The cochlea is air filled
b. The middle ear is fluid filled
c. The ossicles are essential for the structural integrity of the inner ear
d. The tympanic membrane is a dynamic structure
e. The oval window is of larger area than the tympanic membrane

EXPLANATION: THE EAR

The **ear** is made up of **three main parts** – the **outer ear**, the **middle ear** (an air-filled structure) and the **inner ear** (a fluid-filled structure). Sound waves pass through the **external auditory meatus** where they cause the **tympanic membrane** (eardrum) to vibrate.

The **malleolus** bone rests on the tympanic membrane in the middle ear and transmits the sound vibrations through the other tiny inner ear bones (**ossicles**) to the **oval window** on the other side of the middle ear. The tympanic membrane has a larger area than the oval window, so the force transmitted to the oval window is much greater per unit area (15–20 times greater). Basically, this amplifies the vibrations from the tympanic membrane. The amount of energy transmitted to the oval window can be modulated by very small skeletal muscles which alter the **tension** of the **tympanic** membrane and the **ossicles**.

The **oval window** is the gateway to the inner ear. Its vibration **displaces fluid** in the **cochlea** which triggers firing from the sensitive hearing receptor cells – the **hair cells**. The inner ear is made up of the cochlea and the semicircular canal (see pages 93 and 97).

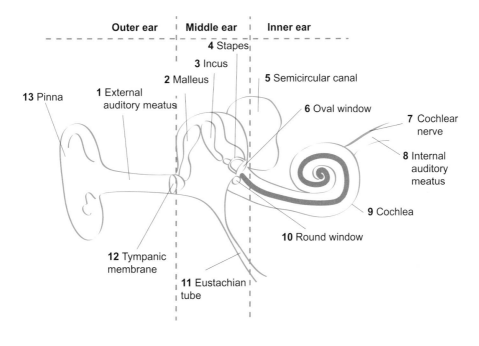

Outer ear | Middle ear | Inner ear

4 Stapes
3 Incus
2 Malleus
5 Semicircular canal
13 Pinna
1 External auditory meatus
6 Oval window
7 Cochlear nerve
8 Internal auditory meatus
9 Cochlea
10 Round window
12 Tympanic membrane
11 Eustachian tube

Answers
30. 1 – B, 2 – E, 3 – I, 4 – F, 5 – D, 6 – H, 7 – M, 8 – A, 9 – J, 10 – K, 11 – C, 12 – L, 13 – G
31. F F F T F

32. In the auditory system

    a. The scala vestibuli has a high concentration of K^+ ions
    b. The spiral ganglion contains cell bodies from the cochlear nerve
    c. Auditory information from one ear is sent to both auditory cortices
    d. Neurotransmitter is released from the bases of hair cells
    e. The organ of Corti is surrounded by perilymph

33. In the auditory system

    a. Sound waves enter the scala vestibuli
    b. The cochlear duct is not influenced by sound waves
    c. Vibration of the basilar membrane varies according to its thickness
    d. The cochlea is a helical structure
    e. The cochlea gives rise to the vestibular nerve

34. Label the transverse section of the cochlea using the options given

Options

    A. Scala vestibuli   B. Cochlear duct
    C. Scala tympani   D. Cochlear nerve
    E. Spiral ganglion   F. Organ of Corti

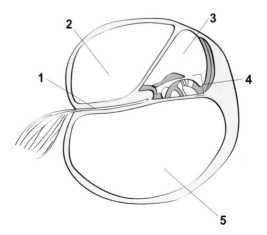

K^+, potassium ion, Na^+, sodium ion

EXPLANATION: THE INNER EAR (i)

Perilymph has a **high concentration of Na⁺**, **endolymph** has a **high concentration of K⁺**. To remember the constituent fluid in the three chambers think **PEP** (perilymph, endolymph, perilymph).

The **organ of Corti** is the important sensory structure in the inner ear – it is situated in the **cochlear duct** and is hence bathed in endolymph. Sound waves travel from the oval window into the **scala vestibuli**, travel along the coiled length of the cochlea and back around the other way through the **scala tympani** until they reach the round window – this structure helps absorb the vibrations and prevents damage to the cochlea. The structure of the cochlea is illustrated below.

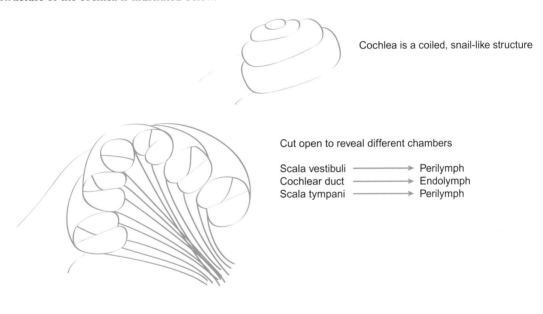

Cochlea is a coiled, snail-like structure

Cut open to reveal different chambers

Scala vestibuli ⟶ Perilymph
Cochlear duct ⟶ Endolymph
Scala tympani ⟶ Perilymph

35. Label the structure below

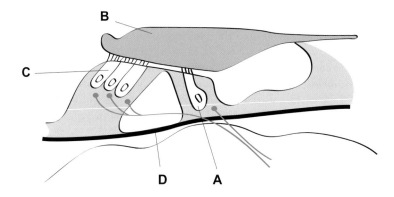

E. State which part of the ear it is found in
F. Briefly explain its role

36. What auditory structures are responsible for

A. Passive frequency discrimination
B. Active frequency discrimination
C. Conducting action potentials to the brainstem
D. Detection of high frequency sounds

EXPLANATION: THE INNER EAR (ii)

The diagram in question 35 is the organ of Corti, which is located in the inner ear **(35E)**.

Transmission of sound energy through the fluid of the inner ear (perilymph and endolymph) causes the **basilar membrane** to **vibrate**. The cochlear receptors (the **inner (35A)** and **outer hair cells (35C)**) mounted on the basilar membrane **(35D)** move with the membrane – the bases of their **cilia** are attached to the **reticular lamina** – a rigid plate. The ends of the outer hair cell cilia attach to the **tectorial membrane (35B)**, but those of the inner hair cell do not quite reach. The resulting 'bending' of the cilia when the basilar membrane vibrates causes an increase in permeability of the hair cell to Na^+, the influx of Na^+ causing depolarization of the cell membrane and transmission of an impulse to the **spiral ganglion** and then to the **auditory nerve (35F)**.

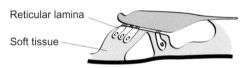

The inner ear at rest

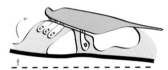

Vibration of the basilar membrane causes bending of cilia

The **basal end** of the **basilar membrane** is **thicker** than the apical end – the **greater energy** in a **high frequency sound** is able to make this part of the membrane vibrate. Lower frequency sounds only have enough energy to make the thinner opposite end of the basilar membrane (the apical end) vibrate, therefore the shape of the basilar membrane can 'sort' different frequencies – this is also known as **passive** (i.e. there is no input from any neurons etc.) **frequency discrimination**.

The outer hair cells are thought to further modulate sound waves as it has been shown in laboratory animals that individual hair cells separated from the basilar membrane respond to stimulation at specific frequencies.

Similarities and differences between inner and outer hair cells

Inner hair cells	Outer hair cells
Glutamate neurotransmitter	Glutamate neurotransmitter
Synapse with afferent fibres only	Synapse with afferent and efferent fibres
High threshold	Low threshold

Answers
35. A – Inner hair cells, B – Tectorial membrane, C – Outer hair cells, D – Basilar membrane, E – This structure makes up part of the inner ear, F – See explanation.
36. A – The basilar membrane, B – outer hair cells, C – The cochlear nerve, D – The basal component of the basilar membrane.

37. The vestibular system

a. Is involved in hearing
b. Influences posture control
c. May be influenced by 5-hydroxytryptamine (5-HT, serotonin) antagonists
d. Includes an otolith organ which detects changes in angular acceleration
e. Is often involved in motion sickness

38. Consider the vestibular system

a. The labyrinth is made up of two otolith organs
b. The semicircular canals contain perilymph
c. It contains hair cells
d. It sends information to the brain via the cochlear nerve
e. It is sensitive to movement only

39. Damage to the vestibular system can cause

a. Vertigo   b. Nausea
c. Ataxia   d. Psychosis
e. Dysphagia

40. Label this diagram of the vestibular system using the following options

Options

A. Ampulla
B. Saccule
C. Semicircular canal
D. Vestibular nerve
E. Vestibulocochlear nerve

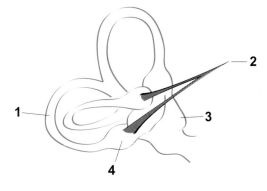

5-HT, 5-hydroxytryptamine (serotonin)

EXPLANATION: THE VESTIBULAR SYSTEM

The **vestibular system** helps control **balance**, **posture** and **eye movements** by sending information on **position**. The vestibular system consists of two main parts:

1. The **labyrinth**: two otolith organs (the **utricle** and **sacculus**) which send information on static head position and linear acceleration.
2. The **semicircular canals**: three rounded tubes each with an **ampulla** which sends information on angular acceleration of the head in a different plane.

The otolith organs and ampullae all contain **endolymph** and **hair cells**. On moving, **inertia** causes the stereocilia to move, which in turn **transduces** a signal. Nerve fibres from the hair cells have their cell bodies in **Scarpa's ganglion** and travel via the vestibular part of **cranial nerve VIII** to the brainstem where they synapse at the vestibular nuclear complex. Fibres are sent from here to cranial nerve nuclei **III**, **IV**, **VI**, the cerebellum and the thalamus, amongst other locations, through a complex series of nuclei. Pathways of the vestibular system are shown below.

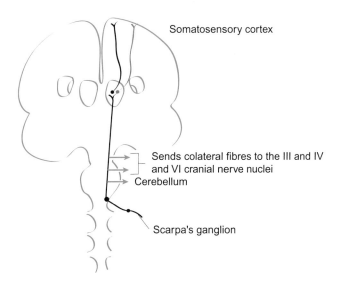

Somatosensory cortex

Sends colateral fibres to the III and IV and VI cranial nerve nuclei

Cerebellum

Scarpa's ganglion

Damage to the vestibular system can cause **nausea**, **vertigo**, **ataxia** and **nystagmus**. The **anticholinergic** drug **hyoscine** or **antihistamines** may be used for the **treatment** of vertigo and nausea. Many drugs may cause nausea and vomiting – opiates and 5-HT antagonists to name but a few.

Answers
37. F T T F T
38. T F T F T
39. T T T F F
40. 1 – C, 2 – D, 3 – B, 4 – A

41. Use the options from the list given to complete the following paragraph

Options

A. Internal capsule
B. Gracile
C. Cuneate
D. Discriminative touch and proprioception
E. Pain and temperature
F. Crude touch and proprioception
G. Lemniscus
H. Dorsal horn
I. Ventral horn
J. Dorsal root ganglion
K. Ventral root ganglion
L. Thalamus
M. Substantia nigra
N. Motor cortex
O. Somatosensory cortex
P. Ascending
Q. Descending
R. Lateral
S. Nerve endings

The somatosensory pathways are important (1) pathways. They carry (2) sensory information from the periphery. In the leg for instance, a stimulus is detected in the periphery by specially adapted (3) and travels towards the spinal cord along a pseudobipolar nerve fibre – the cell body of which is located in the (4). The axon enters the spinal cord and ascends along the (5) fasciculus until it terminates upon synapsing with the (6) nucleus. From here, fibres swing around anteriorly as internal arcuate fibres and decussate to form the medial (7). They continue to ascend and on reaching the diencephalon, synapse in the ventral posterior nucleus of the (8). Cell bodies here send out afferent fibres which travel up through the (9) and terminate in the (10).

42. Label the diagram showing the topographical relationships of the primary somatosensory cortex, using the options given

Options

A. Hand
B. Genitals
C. Leg
D. Lips

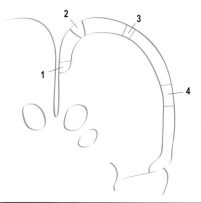

EXPLANATION: SOMATOSENSORY PATHWAYS

The **somatosensory system** is concerned with the **sensations** of **touch**, **pain**, **temperature** and **proprioception** – in fact, any sensation we are aware of. Sensory information is sent to the **somatosensory cortex** where parts of the body are mapped out to form a sensory homunculus (see also 'motor homunculus' page 119). If the size of areas devoted to sensation in the brain are mapped out as an anatomical likeness of a human, we can see that particularly sensitive parts of the body such as the **fingertips**, **lips** and **tongue** have more cortical space devoted to them than the trunk or legs.

The somatosensory pathways are shown in the diagram below.

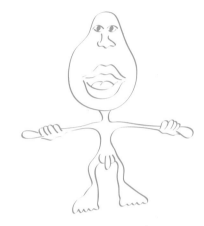

Sensory homunculus

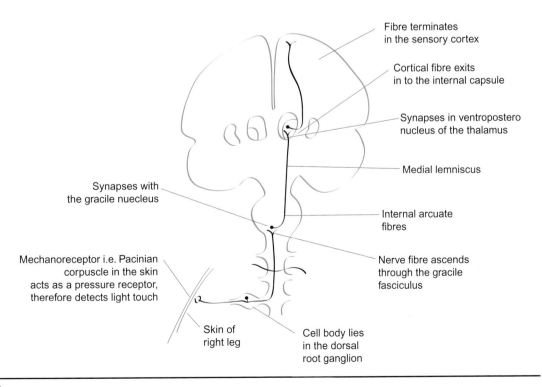

Fibre terminates in the sensory cortex

Cortical fibre exits in to the internal capsule

Synapses in ventropostero nucleus of the thalamus

Medial lemniscus

Synapses with the gracile nuecleus

Internal arcuate fibres

Mechanoreceptor i.e. Pacinian corpuscle in the skin acts as a pressure receptor, therefore detects light touch

Nerve fibre ascends through the gracile fasciculus

Skin of right leg

Cell body lies in the dorsal root ganglion

Answers
41. 1 – P, 2 – D, 3 – S, 4 – J, 5 – B, 6 – B, 7 – G, 8 – L, 9 – A, 10 – O
42. 1 – B, 2 – C, 3 – A, 4 – D

43. Study the diagram of the somatosensory pathways below

A. What would be the effect of a large lesion here?
B. What would be the effect of a hemi-cordotomy here?
C. Which nucleus is this?
D. What is this part of the somatosensory pathway called?

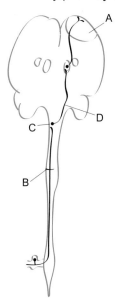

44. Consider skin receptors

a. There are one or two types of receptor found only in the skin
b. Pacinian corpuscles are unencapsulated fibres
c. Peritrichal nerve endings are found in glabrous skin
d. Pain and temperature sensation is detected by encapsulated fibres
e. Ruffini endings detect pressure and stretch modalities

EXPLANATION: SOMATOSENSORY PATHWAYS AND SKIN RECEPTORS

Damage to the **somatosensory cortex** or the pathways supplying it causes **loss** of **touch**, **pain**, **temperature** and **proprioceptive sensation** (anaesthesia). The location and the extent of the sensory loss depends on the site of the lesion. **43A**: If the entire **somatosensory cortex** was **damaged** there would be gross sensory deficit on the **contralateral** side of the body, including the **face**, **arms** and **legs**. A smaller focal lesion would only affect specific parts of the body according to the site of the lesion in the cortex. A lesion to the spinal cord at **43B** would cause ipsilateral sensory loss below the T8/9 level (approximately).

The other important structures in the somatosensory pathway here are the **gracile nucleus** (**43C**) and the medial lemniscus (**43D**)

There are a variety of **receptors** in the skin for **discriminative touch**, **light touch**, **vibration**, **pain** and **temperature**. They are divided into two groups – **encapsulated** (nerve endings associated with non-neural cell types which modify their function) i.e. **Pacinian corpuscles** and **Meissner's corpuscles** and **unencapsulated** (bare nerve endings) i.e. **C fibres** which transmit pain and temperature information. The distribution of skin receptors varies according to skin type – glabrous (hairless) skin versus hairy skin.

Structure	Sensitive to	Found in
Pacinian corpuscles	Vibration	Hairy and glabrous skin
Meissner's corpuscles	Tactile stimuli	Glabrous skin only
Merkel endings	Tactile stimuli	Hairy and glabrous skin
Ruffini endings	Pressure and stretch	Hairy and glabrous skin
Peritrichal nerve endings	Light touch	Hairy skin only

The different skin receptors are shown below.

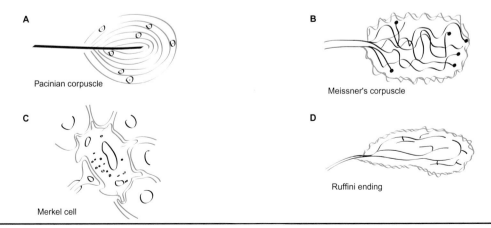

A

Pacinian corpuscle

B

Meissner's corpuscle

C

Merkel cell

D

Ruffini ending

Answers
43. See explanation
44. F F F F T

45. Match the feature in the numbered list with the peripheral nerve fibres given in the options below

Options

A. A-beta fibres
C. C fibres
E. A-delta fibres

B. C and A-beta fibres
D. A-alpha, A-beta and A-delta fibres
F. A-alpha fibres

1. Unmyelinated
2. Sensory, from Golgi tendon organs
3. Somatic motor
4. Sensory, from hair follicles, carry pain and temperature information
5. Carry pain and temperature information

46. Receptive fields

a. Are only found in particularly sensitive areas of skin
b. Are each supplied by a single nerve fibre
c. May be influenced by interneurons
d. Involve nerve fibres with many end-terminals
e. Involve nerve fibres that are not influenced by their neighbours

EXPLANATION: SKIN RECEPTORS

Type C fibres are the only fibres in the list that are unmyelinated – the rest have a myelin sheath. Diameter and conduction velocity are proportional to one-another and increase in the following way:

- Smallest diameter and slowest conduction velocity – C fibres
- Largest diameter and fastest conduction velocity – A-delta, A-gamma, A-beta and A-alpha

C fibres have **unencapsulated nerve endings** and signal **pain** and **temperature** information. **A-delta fibres** carry **pain**, **temperature** and **sensory** information from hair follicles. **A-gamma fibres** have a **motor** role in muscle spindles. **A-beta fibres** carry sensory information from skin receptors – type Ib from Golgi tendon organs and type II from muscle spindles (in muscle), Meissner's and Pacinian corpuscles and larger hair follicles. **A-delta fibres** are **motor neurons** and supply skeletal muscle.

A **receptive field** is an area of skin supplied by a single **sensory nerve fibre**. The receptive fields of **many sensory fibres overlap** which helps accurately localize the stimulus. The degree of firing is influenced by **lateral inhibition** via **inhibitory interneurons** – the receptive field which contains the bulk of the stimulus has a firing rate of the greatest magnitude – this overcomes the inhibitory influence of the interneurons (EPSP > IPSP). Receptive fields containing only part of the stimulus fire weakly and are easily inhibited (EPSP < IPSP). This is shown in diagrammatic form below.

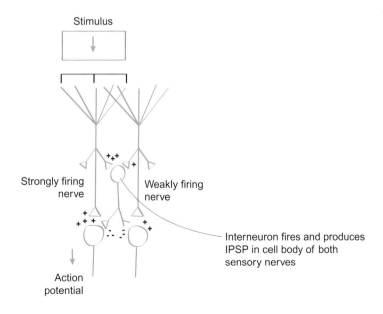

47. Nociceptors

a. Are not found in the viscera
b. Are mostly composed of free nerve endings
c. Pain may be transmitted by both delta and C fibres
d. C fibres are responsible for the fast component of pain transduction
e. Transduction may be mediated by numerous inflammatory mediators

48. The following are all chemical mediators in the perception of pain

a. Bradykinin
b. Prostaglandins
c. Substance P
d. Neuropeptide Y
e. Histamine

49. What is sensitization? Name three factors that can induce sensitization of nociceptive primary sensory neurones.

50. Opioids

A–C. List three brain areas that have a high level of opioid peptides and receptors
D. Briefly explain how morphine acting at these sites produces analgesia.

51. Opioids

a. Cause constipation
b. Cause respiratory depression
c. Cause mydriasis (pupillary dilatation)
d. May cause nausea and vomiting
e. Include diamorphine, codeine and methadone

Ca^{2+}, calcium ion; CNS, central nervous system; GABA, gamma-aminobutyric acid; K^+, potassium ion, NRM, nucleus raphe magnus; NRPG, nucleus reticularis paragiganticellularis; PAG, periaqueductal grey

EXPLANATION: NOCICEPTION

Pain is defined as an **unpleasant sensory** or **emotional experience** with actual or potential tissue damage. The scientific term for pain is **nociception**.

Nociceptors are found in **skin**, the **viscera**, **skeletal** and **cardiac muscle**. There are two types of histological pain fibre. **A-delta fibres** (myelinated) and **C fibres** (unmyelinated). The A-delta fibres are faster conductors of pain signals than the C fibres. If you hit your thumb with a hammer you will feel two components to the pain sensation (don't try it!): the sharp instantaneous pain as your thumb is hit, and a second dull throbbing type of pain that follows. The former is due to the fast conduction of pain by the delta fibres, the latter due to the slower conduction by the C fibres.

Chemical or **inflammatory mediators** modulate the activity of the nociceptors and play an important role in pain conduction. **Bradykinin**, **histamine**, **serotonin** and **prostaglandins** play a role in sensitization of the nociceptor and surrounding tissue. **Substance P** is a neurotransmitter in the spinal cord which is an important component of the pain pathway. **Neuropeptide Y** does not appear to have a role in the perception of pain; however, it is known to be a neurotransmitter in the sympathetic nervous system. **Sensitization** follows tissue damage to the area around a wound and **lowers** the **threshold** needed to depolarize the nerve ending. This causes the tissue to become hypersensitive to pain (hyperalgesia) **(49)**.

EXPLANATION: PHARMACOLOGY OF PAIN

High levels of opioid peptides and receptors are found in the **periaqueductal grey**, the **nucleus raphe magnus**, the **nucleus reticularis paragiganticellularis** and the **dorsal horn** of the spinal cord (especially the **substantia gelatinosia**) **(50A–C)**.

In the PAG, NRM and NRPG **opioids inhibit** the **release of GABA** which reduces inhibition of the **descending serotonergic pathway**. This reduces the transmission of nociceptive signals through the dorsal horn of the spinal cord. The dorsal horn is targeted directly by opioids which inhibit the **firing** of projecting neurons and neurotransmitter release **(50D)**.

There are three types of opioid receptor in the CNS:

Receptor	Effects	
delta (δ)	Increase K$^+$ permeability	Inhibit adenylate cyclase
mu (μ)	Increase K$^+$ permeability	Inhibit adenylate cyclase
kappa (κ)	Decrease Ca^{2+} permeability	Inhibit adenylate cyclase

Opioids are **central depressants** and cause many side-effects. In the gut, **morphine** acts on mu receptors and **slows down peristalsis** – this can be useful in patients with diarrhoea. The opioid receptor antagonist **naloxone** can be used to treat patients with **respiratory depression** caused by opioid overdose – other common effects of opioids are **pinpoint pupils**, **itching**, **nausea** and **vomiting**.

Answers
47. F T T T F
48. F T T T F
49. See explanation
50. See explanation
51. T T F T T

52. Consider pain pathways

    a. Signals from the periphery are sent to the ventral horn in the spinal cord
    b. Synapses of pain fibres in the spinal cord often have many inputs
    c. Nociceptive information is carried to the brain by a single pair of tracts
    d. The spinothalamic tract decussates in the medulla
    e. The ascending nociceptive pathways synapse at numerous sites in the central nervous system (CNS)

53. Complete the paragraph below with the most appropriate word from the options given

Each option may be used once, more than once or not at all.

Options

    A. Dorsal horn   **B.** Ventral horn
    C. Thalamus   **D.** Periaqueductal grey
    E. Raphe nucleus   **F.** Rostroventral medulla
    G. C fibres   **H.** gamma fibres
    I. Decussate   **J.** Leave the spinal cord
    K. Spinothalamic tract   **L.** Reticulospinal tract
    M. Descending tract

Following a laceration to the skin delta and (1) send axons to the (2) of the spinal cord where they synapse with numerous other fibres such as those from the (3). These inputs modulate the transmission of nociceptive information from the periphery. Neurons with cell bodies in the (4) send out axons which (5) almost straight away. These axons travel up through the spinal cord through several tracts – the most important one being the (6). This tract terminates at a variety of destinations including the (7), (8), (9) and the (10).

CNS, central nervous system

EXPLANATION: PAIN PATHWAYS

Nociceptive pathways in the CNS are illustrated and explained below.

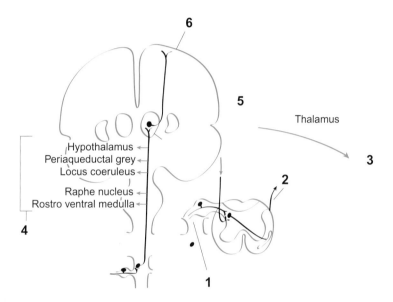

1 Peripheral nociceptive fibre – the cell body is in the dorsal root ganglion (typical of a sensory nerve fibre) and sends a fibre to the dorsal horn

2 There are many inputs into the dorsal horn. Ascending tract (spinothalamic tract decussates here)

3 These inputs modulate nociceptive signals by release of endogenous opioids (known as endorphins and enkephalins) Release of these neurotransmiters inhibits signal transmission in the ascending tracts and reduces the sensation of pain. There are two pairs of spinothalamic tracts-lateral and ventral

4 Fibres from the spinothalamic tract terminate at numerous destinations

5 Descending tract carries regulatory input from higher centres

6 Fibres from the thalamus also terminate at the insula, prefontal coretex and the basal ganglia

54. What is TENS? Briefly explain its physiological basis and how it may be used clinically

55. What is referred pain? What mechanism is likely to underlie this phenomenon?

TENS, transcutaneous electronic nerve stimulation

EXPLANATION: TRANSCUTANEOUS ELECTRONIC NERVE STIMULATION AND REFERRED PAIN

TENS (transcutaneous electronic nerve stimulation) is a means of providing analgesia using **electrodes** placed on the **skin** and applying an **electric current** across it (54).

It is not entirely clear how TENS works, but it is thought that it occurs by stimulation of **A-beta** fibres through the skin. A-beta fibres act by inhibiting **A-beta** neurons which carry nociceptive signals to the brain. It is also thought that TENS may play a role in the **release** of **endogenous opioids**.

TENS may be useful in chronic painful conditions such as musculoskeletal pain, post-surgical pain and acute pain such as labour. It has been found that up to 70 per cent of chronic pain patients initially respond well to TENS but with regular use over one year this figure drops to 30 per cent as tolerance is acquired (54).

Referred pain is a pain sensation **considerably removed** from the **tissues causing the pain**. It frequently originates from one of the **visceral organs** and is referred to an area on the body's surface or a deep part of the body. Many visceral disorders have referred pain as their sole symptom, making knowledge of these phenomena important clinically (55). The localization of referred pain is shown opposite.

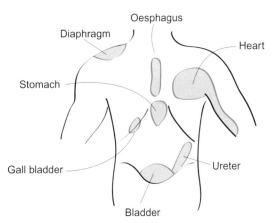

The most likely mechanism for referred pain is through the **synapsing** of **visceral pain fibres** with the same **second-order neurons** that receive pain fibres from the skin. When the visceral pain fibres are stimulated, they trigger the second-order neurons that they 'share' with the skin pain fibres. This gives rise to the sensation of referred pain, which is perceived as arising from the patch of skin innervated by these neurons (55).

There are two types of transmission pathways: the **parietal pathway**, where sensations are conducted directly into the **local spinal nerves** from the **parietal peritoneum** and **pleura** or **pericardium** and the pain is located directly over the affected area, and **true visceral pain** which is transmitted via sensory fibres in the autonomic nervous system, frequently far from the affected organ. True visceral pain is usually localized in the **dermatomal segment** the visceral organ arose from (55).

Answers
54. See explanation
55. See explanation

MOTOR SYSTEMS

MOTOR SYSTEMS

1. Complete the paragraph below from the options given

Options

A. Internal capsule
C. Medial lemniscus
E. Red nucleus and the thalamus
G. Lateral corticospinal tract
I. Ventral corticospinal tract
K. Primary motor
M. Dendrites
O. 85 per cent
Q. 15 per cent
S. Cell bodies
U. Primary motor and sensory

B. Axons
D. Lentiform nucleus and the thalamus
F. Red nucleus
H. Striatum and the pallidum
J. Primary motor and premotor
L. Ventral horns
N. Pyramids
P. 50 per cent
R. Median aperture
T. Sensory

Corticospinal tracts mainly consist of **(1)** which arise in the **(2)** areas of the frontal lobe and the **(3)** area of the parietal lobe. The corticospinal fibres descend through the cerebral cortex and converge to enter the **(4)** which on its journey downward passes between the **(5)**. In the midbrain these fibres exit the **(4)**, continuing down through the crus cerebri. Some fibres terminate at targets in the brainstem such as the pontine nuclei, inferior olivary nucleus and **(6)**. After reaching the inferior portion of the pons, the corticospinal fibres emerge ventrally to form the **(7)**. When the corticospinal fibres reach the inferior portion of the medulla, **(8)** of them decussate to form the **(9)** in the spinal cord. The remainder continue downwards to form the **(10)**. The corticospinal fibres terminate in the **(11)** of the spinal cord where they synapse with motor neurons.

2. Axons from the motor cortex

a. Include axons which terminate on interneurons
b. Include axons which terminate on motor neurons
c. Include 50 per cent which decussate in the medulla
d. Include axons which terminate on lower motor neurons in the brainstem
e. Pass through the crus cerebri

EXPLANATION: THE MOTOR SYSTEM

The **motor system** controls movement, which is either **voluntary** (somatic) or **non-voluntary** such as a reflex. **Voluntary** movements are **planned** out in the **motor cortex**, **supplementary motor cortex** and the **premotor cortex** and executed via the **basal ganglia**.

In the frontal lobe, corticospinal tracts may arise in the primary motor, premotor and supplementary motor areas. They may also arise in the somatosensory cortex in the parietal cortex. The figure below shows the corticospinal tracts.

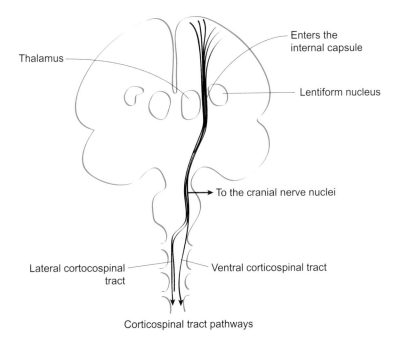

Corticospinal tract pathways

---

3. Consider the diagram of the corticospinal pathways below

A. What would be the effect of a lesion here?
B. Would a lesion here be likely to have a greater or lesser effect than a lesion at A?
C. Explain briefly what is happening here
D What would be the effect of a lesion here? How would it differ from that in A?
E. Which single limb of the body are most of these nerve fibres in D going to?

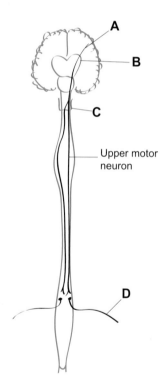

A

B

C

Upper motor
neuron

D

EXPLANATION: CORTICOSPINAL PATHWAYS

A. A **lesion** to the **motor cortex** of one hemisphere (such as in a stroke) will affect the **contralateral** half of the body. The effects are highly variable, depending on which part of the motor cortex is affected. A **small lesion** would normally have a highly **localized** effect – affecting only a small part of the body such as a hand or several fingers. **Larger lesions** affect a greater area of cortex and have a more significant effect on motor function i.e. hemiplegia. A **neuron** that arises in the **cortex** is known as an upper motor neuron – damage to one of these fibres is called an upper motor neuron lesion.

B. The **fibres** that pass through the **internal capsule** are highly condensed and occupy a relatively small area. An internal capsule lesion therefore has the potential to wipe out a very high proportion of the axons carried in a tract. For this reason, a lesion here is likely to cause a much **greater loss** of **function**.

C. This shows the **pyramids** and is the point where part of the **corticospinal tract decussates**; 85 per cent of these fibres cross over to form the **lateral corticospinal** tract, the remainder carry on downwards forming the **ventral corticospinal** tract.

D. **Lower motor neurons** have their cell bodies in the **ventral horn** of the spinal cord. Damage to one of these fibes produces a lower motor neuron injury. The comparison between upper and lower motor neuron injuries is shown below:

Upper motor neuron	Lower motor neuron
Muscle spasticity	Muscle flaccidity
Relatively normal muscle bulk	Muscle wasting
Brisk tendon reflexes	Absent tendon reflexes
Recovery unlikely	Some possibility of recovery

Lower motor neuron injuries are likely to occur if the muscle or nerve directly supplying it are cut, or if the cell body of the motor neuron is attacked by a pathogen such as the polio virus. Upper motor neuron injuries are commonly seen as a result of stroke. This is discussed in more detail on the next page.

E. The majority of these fibres are supplying the left leg.

Answers
3. See explanation

4. **Match the tracts in the numbered list which occur in one half of the spinal cord with the best description**

Options

A. Corticospinal
C. Reticulospinal
E. Vestibulospinal

B. Corticobulbar
D. Tectospinal

1. Pair of tracts which arise in the pons and medulla. They are thought to aid co-ordination of movement
2. A single tract whose fibres arise ipsilaterally and that is concerned with the maintenance of upright posture
3. Pair of tracts – one ipsilateral and one contralateral – carrying information on fine motor control
4. Fibres from this tract supply the cranial nerves
5. A tract arising contralaterally in the tectum that influences control of neurons in the neck

5. **Damage to a lower motor neuron may cause**

a. Flaccid paralysis
b. Loss of stretch reflex
c. Muscle atrophy
d. Tremor
e. Muscle spasticity

6. **Damage to an upper motor neuron may cause**

a. Flaccid paralysis
b. Exaggerated stretch reflexes
c. Muscle atrophy
d. The clasp knife reflex
e. Muscle spasticity

MCQ, multiple choice question

EXPLANATION: MOTOR PATHWAYS

Lower motor neurons synapse directly with **skeletal muscle**. Without their input the muscle will be in a **permanently relaxed** state (**flaccid**) and will atrophy. Tremor is unlikely since there are no motor neurons to activate the muscle fibres – consequently the stretch reflex is lost too. See the figure on page 123 for more information on this pathway.

In contrast, damage to an **upper motor neuron** leaves the muscle with its lower motor neuron supply intact. The lower motor neuron still influences the muscle – **loss** of **inhibitory descending fibres** means the lower motor neuron remains active. Consequently the muscle is in a contracted state (it is described as being 'spastic') – not flaccid. The loss of the inhibitory descending fibres causes an **exaggerated stretch reflex**. The **clasp knife reflex** may be seen when proximal muscle groups like the biceps in the arm are in a contracted state – if the forearm is extended, tension is increased until a certain point is reached when the muscle relaxes transiently to allow the arm to extend fully. This is due to the **golgi tendon organs** in the muscle tendons responding to the **increase** in **tension** on the muscle and their reflex inhibition of the motor neurons.

This is a hard question but it is useful to have a knowledge of these tracts for more difficult MCQs. The corticospinal tract is the most important of all these pathways.

The vestibulospinal tract is easy enough to remember because the vestibular system is involved in control of balance and posture. Anything with 'bulbar' in it is related to the brainstem – hence the connection with the cranial nerves.

Answers
4. 1 – C, 2 – E, 3 – A, 4 – B, 5 – D
5. T T T F F
6. F T F T T

7. Match the motor modality with its location on the motor cortex shown below

Options

A. Thumb
B. Foot
C. Hip
D. Tongue
E. Arm
F. Hand
G. Leg
H. Fingers

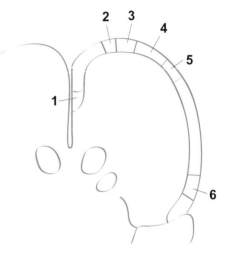

8. Which part of the brain provides voluntary control of muscle?

A. Thalamus
B. Hypothalamus
C. Medulla
D. Pons
E. Cerebral cortex

9. The motor cortex

A. Contains higher centres for control of movement on the ipsilateral side of the body
B. Gives rise to a large proportion of the pyramidal tracts
C. Sends fibres that synapse with motor neurons and other neuron types
D. Is also known as the striate cortex because of its striped appearance
E. Contains a motor homunculus

EXPLANATION: TOPOGRAPHICAL REPRESENTATION OF THE MOTOR SYSTEM (THE MOTOR HOMUNCULUS)

While Brodmann mapped out the cellular architecture of the cerebral cortex, Sherrington and Penfield found that in the motor and somatosensory cortices, **parts of the body** were **represented by specific regions** on the surface of the brain. Some parts of the body have a disproportionately large representation depending on which cortex they are in – these representations can be mapped out diagramatically as a **motor homunculus** (or in the somatosensory cortex a sensory homunculus – see page 99). The **motor cortex** devotes **more space** to areas of the body that deal with **fine movement,** such as the fingers, thumbs and hands, and some of the facial muscles such as those in the lips and tongue – this is represented in the motor homunculus shown below.

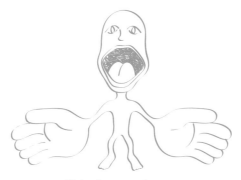

Motor homunculus
Note disproportionate sizes of fingers,
lips and thumbs

Centres controlling **voluntary movements** are found in the **motor cortex** on the **contralateral** side of the body they control – the **pyramidal tracts (corticospinal)** mostly arise here, **decussating** at the **pyramids** – these fibres synapse with **motor neurons** and **spinal interneurons**. The visual cortex has a striped appearance and is sometimes described as the striate cortex (this does not apply to the rest of the occipital cortex, of which the visual cortex is a part). As in the somatosensory cortex, the motor cortex also contains a **homunculus** (in both hemispheres) – a **topographical representation** of the **human body**.

10. Consider the basal ganglia

    a. They are primarily concerned with sensation
    b. The corpus striatum is composed of the caudate nucleus and pallidum
    c. The striatum, subthalamic nucleus and substantia nigra receive inhibitory afferents from the cerebral cortex
    d. Dopaminergic neurons in the substantia nigra excite and inhibit striatal neurons
    e. The major output of the striatum is inhibitory and to the pallidum

11. Consider the connections of the basal ganglia

    a. The caudate and putamen receive only a small proportion of their inputs from the motor cortex
    b. The main output of the lentiform nucleus is to the pallidum
    c. The substantia nigra and basal ganglia have reciprocal connections
    d. The main output of the globus pallidus is to the thalamus
    e. None of the above are true

12. The corpus striatum is best described as the

    a. Caudate, putamen and globus pallidus
    b. Internal capsule and its contents
    c. Globus pallidus and putamen only
    d. Thalamus and the ventroposterior nucleus
    e. Caudate and putamen only

13. The lentiform nucleus is composed of the

    a. Substantia nigra and the nigrostriatal tract
    b. Caudate and the putamen
    c. Globus pallidus and putamen
    d. Amygdala and the tail of the caudate nucleus
    e. Thalamus and the substantia nigra

EXPLANATION: THE BASAL GANGLIA

The **basal ganglia** are a collection of anatomical structures in the midbrain responsible for **movement** and include the **corpus striatum**, **subthalamic nucleus** and **substantia nigra**.

The corpus striatum is made up of the **striatum** (**caudate nucleus** and **putamen**) and the **pallidum** – these two components have important functional roles in the control of movement.

The **striatum**, **subthalamic nucleus** and **substantia nigra** all receive excitatory signals from the cerebral cortex. The **major output** of the **striatum to the pallidum** is **inhibitory**. At rest the striatum is inhibited, leaving the **pallidum** to exert its **inhibitory effects** on the **thalamus**. On movement, the **striatum** is activated and **inhibits** the **pallidum**. This permits **excitation** of the **thalamus** and, in turn, the **cortex**. The connections of the basal ganglia are illustrated below.

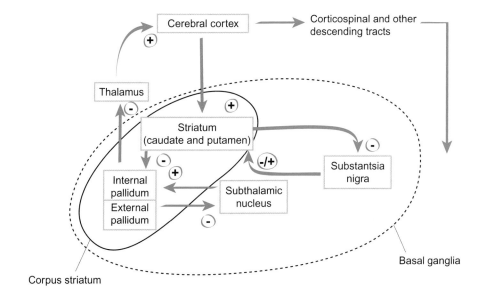

14. In the somatic muscle the stretch reflex

    a. Is not influenced by the central nervous system (CNS)
    b. Is a monosynaptic reflex
    c. Is mediated by acetylcholine (ACh) in the muscle
    d. May lead to inhibition of antagonist muscles
    e. Is often exaggerated after a stroke or upper motor neurone injury

15. What neuronal circuit does the diagram below illustrate? Complete the diagram by filling in the missing labels

Options

    A. Ia afferent fibre
    B. Ib afferent fibre
    C. Motor neuron
    D. Muscle spindle
    E. Inhibitory interneuron
    F. Tendon organ

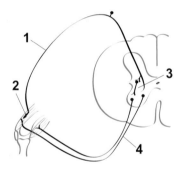

16. Label the diagram of a muscle spindle below

Options

    A. Nuclear bag fibre
    B. Nuclear chain fibre
    C. Capsule
    D. Motor nerve fibres
    E. Primary sensory endings
    F. Secondary sensory endings
    G. Motor endings
    H. Sensory nerve fibres

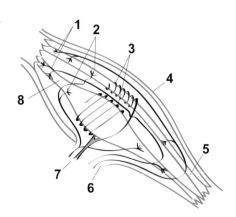

ACh, acetylcholine; CNS, central nervous system

EXPLANATION: THE STRETCH REFLEX

Descending fibres may synapse in the spinal cord and **influence** the **stretch reflex**. A stroke or other neurological insult often destroys **upper motor neurons** which may play a role in **damping down** this reflex. Their loss produces an **exaggerated stretch** reflex – typically described clinically as a '**brisk**' response to a stimulus such as a tendon tap with a neurological hammer.

The diagram illustrates a polysynaptic stretch reflex arc (15).

Muscle spindles are proprioceptive organs (they act as **stretch** detectors. responding to changes in muscle length) along with **Golgi tendon organs** (which act as **tension** detectors and, as their name suggests, are found in tendons). The **spindle** is formed by a **fibrous capsule** and contains thin muscle fibres known as **intrafusal fibres**, described as either nuclear bag fibres or nuclear chain fibres according to their shape (the bulkier muscle fibres outside the spindle are termed **extrafusal** fibres). The spindle is supplied by two afferent (sensory) fibres A-alpha or Ia which form primary sensory endings and A-beta or type II fibres which form secondary sensory endings. The motor supply to the intrafusal fibres comes from A-gamma nerve fibres.

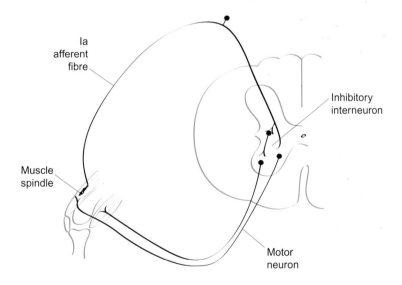

Ia afferent fibre

Inhibitory interneuron

Muscle spindle

Motor neuron

Stretch of the **muscle** initiates the **polysynaptic reflex arc** (tendon jerk reflex).

Answers
14. F T T T T
15. 1 – A, 2 – D, 3 – E, 4 – C
16. 1 – G, 2 – F, 3 – E, 4 – C, 5 – B, 6 – H, 7 – D, 8 – A

17. Cerebellar lesions

a. Are normally contralateral to any resulting motor defect
b. Usually only cause nystagmus if localized in the vermis
c. Are rare in alcoholics
d. May cause a tremor
e. Cause muscle spasticity

18. Consider cerebellar lesion

A. List two postural deficits that might be seen in a patient with a cerebellar lesion
B. List two voluntary movement deficits that might be seen in a patient with a cerebellar lesion

19. Nystagmus

a. Is an oscillating movement of the eye
b. Is unusual in neurological disease
c. Implies pathology in the vestibular system, the cerebellum or brainstem
d. Cannot be induced clinically
e. Has slow and fast phases

20. Damage to the cerebellum

a. May cause nystgamus when looking to one side
b. Causes tremor
c. Motor defects are ipsilateral to the lesion
d. Can make repeated rapid movements difficult
e. Causes muscle spasticity

EXPLANATION: MOVEMENT DISORDERS (i)

Cerebellar **nystagmus** is caused by a lesion in the midline (**vermis**) of the cerebellum. It describes **repetitive flicking movements** of the eyes in one plane of movement when the eyes move to one side. This is normally in the horizontal plane, the vertical plane of eye movements is less commonly affected. Degeneration of the vermis may occur in **chronic alcoholism** causing **tremor**, an unsteady, staggering wide-based **ataxic gait**, **swaying** from side to side and nystagmus. Lesions in the cerebellum do not cause muscle spasticity. Other signs seen in patients with a damaged cerebellum are: **dysmetria** – poorly co-ordinated movements when reaching out for an object – **adiadochokinesis** – inability to make fast repetitive movements such as touching the palm of one hand with the palm and then back of the other hand rapidly – and **dysarthria** – slurring speech.

Loss of balance when standing erect with feet together and eyes closed (**Romberg's sign**) and a wide-based stance are seen in patients with a cerebellar lesion (**18A**). Voluntary movement deficits that might be seen are a broad-based and staggering gait, jerky, conjugate eye movements and irregular, explosive and slurring speech (**18B**).

Nystagmus can be induced in normal individuals by tilting the head slightly forward and rotating the patient about ten times in a revolving chair. When stopped, the endolymph in the lateral and horizontal semicircular canals of the vestibular system continues moving and induces nystagmus for about 30 seconds. Nystagmus has slow and fast phases – in the case of post-rotatory nystagmus the fast component is in the opposite direction to the direction of rotation.

Answers
17. F T F T F
18. See explanation
19. T F T F T
20. T T T T F

21. Consider dyskinesias

a. A dyskinesia usually includes sensory loss
b. A dyskinesia may affect facial and tongue movements and swallowing
c. Choreiform movements are irregular, brisk and jerky
d. Tremor is characterized by regularly alternating movements of small amplitude
e. Ballism is an exaggerated form of athetoid movement

22. The following are associated with Parkinson's disease

a. Micrographia
b. Shuffling gait
c. Resting tremor
d. Tremor on movement
e. Frozen immobile face

23. Which of the following is NOT a symptom of Parkinson's disease

a. 'Mask-like facial expression'
b. Intention tremor
c. Tremor at rest
d. Bradykinesia
e. Cog-wheel rigidity

24. Parkinson's disease

a. Is usually not treatable
b. Is fatal
c. Is usually caused by degeneration of neurons in the thalamus
d. Is characterized by a resting tremor, bradykinesia and rigidity
e. Usually has an onset in early age

25. Disorders confined to the basal ganglia include

a. Ballism
b. Alzheimer's disease
c. Huntington's disease
d. Parkinson's disease
e. Korsakoff's syndrome

CNS, central nervous system

EXPLANATION: MOVEMENT DISORDERS (ii)

A **dyskinesia** is an **improper movement** and not directly related to sensory loss. It may affect any part of the body with a **somatic motor supply** and is most striking in movement disorders conditions such as **Parkinson's disease** and **Huntington's chorea**. **Ballism** is an **exaggerated** form of **choreiform movement** which causes the limbs to fling around uncontrollably. The condition **hemiballismus** is caused by **damage** to the **subthalamic nucleus** and, as its name suggests, affects one side of the body. **Athetoid** movements are irregular, slow and sinuous. The typical appearance of a patient with Parkinson's disease is illustrated below.

Ballism (unco-ordinated flinging movements of the body) results from damage to the **subthalamic nucleus** – a ventral part of the thalamus (**hemiballismus** is the same type of disorder, but confined to one half of the body).

Alzheimer's disease is characterized by **cortical neuronal loss** of **cholinergic neurons** –some are **lost** from the **basal ganglia** but these are only a small fraction of those lost from the entire brain.

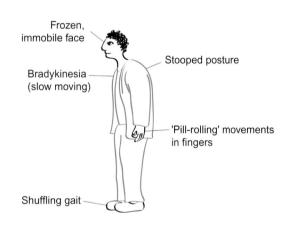

Frozen, immobile face

Stooped posture

Bradykinesia (slow moving)

'Pill-rolling' movements in fingers

Shuffling gait

Huntington's disease is caused by loss of neurons in the **cerebral cortex** and the **striatum**.

Parkinson's disease is caused by degeneration of **dopaminergic neurons** in the **nigrostriatal tract** which starts in the midbrain.

The **mediodorsal thalamic nucleus** shows degenerative changes in **Korsakoff's syndrome**, but the thalamus is not part of the basal ganglia. Mammillary body haemorrhage is another feature of Korsakoff's syndrome.

Micrographia is small writing characteristic of the disease when patients are asked to write sentences in clinic – this is also seen in people on anti-psychotic medications, some of which act by inhibiting dopamine receptors in the CNS causing Parkinson-like symptoms (Parkinsonism). Tremor induced by movement is not characteristic of Parkinson's disease.

Answers
21. F T T T F
22. T T T F T
23. F T F F F
24. F F F T F
25. T F T T F

26. Parkinsonism may be induced by the following drugs

a. Codeine

b. Haloperidol

c. Bromocriptine

d. ʟ-Dopa

e. Imipramine

27. In Parkinson's disease anticholinergic drugs are used to treat the following symptoms

a. Rigidity

b. Pill-rolling movements

c. Tremor

d. Shuffling gait

e. Bradykinesia

28. Chorea is

a. Not known to have a genetic cause

b. Always bilateral when present

c. Caused by Huntington's disease

d. Caused by damage to the primary motor cortex

e. Characterized by slow, repetitive movements

29. The following are features of Huntington's disease

a. Chorea

b. It is an autosomal dominant condition

c. It can be treated by risperidone

d. There is cell death in the cerebral cortex and the thalamus

e. Dementia

30. Huntington's chorea

a. Is inherited in an autosomally dominant fashion

b. Typically onsets in late life

c. Does not cause mental deterioration

d. Typically involves loss of neurons in the striatum that leads to choreiform movements

e. Has a good prognosis

EXPLANATION: MOVEMENT DISORDERS (iii)

Haloperidol is a dopamine antagonist (thus mimicking the effects of a dopamine deficiency) and is used as an antipsychotic drug. **Codeine** is an opioid commonly used as an analgesic – side-effects include addiction, stomach bleeding, constipation, constricted pupils and kidney and liver damage. **Bromocriptine** is a dopamine agonist – it is used as an anti-Parkinsonian drug as is L-dopa (levadopa). **Imipramine** is a tricyclic antidepressant whose common side-effects include constipation, dry mouth, cardiac arrhythmias and drowsiness.

Huntington's chorea usually manifests between the ages of 30 and 50 years. It causes neuronal loss – most marked in the striatum – which leads to **progressive mental deterioration** and choreiform movements. Huntingdon's chorea is a **chronic degenerative condition** for which there is **no effective treatment or cure** – the condition is **fatal** typically 15 to 20 years from diagnosis. The **autosomal dominant** nature of the disease means that an affected parent has a 50 per cent chance of passing it onto his or her offspring which brings up the difficult personal issue of screening children of affected adults.

Answers
26. F T F F F
27. T F F F F
28. F F T F F
29. T T F T T
30. T F F T F

SECTION 5

COGNITION

1. Which of the following are true?

a. Frontal lobe lesions often give rise to high level cognitive disorders
b. Lesions in Wernicke's area result in aphasia
c. For the majority of left-handers, the left hemisphere is dominant for language functions
d. Right parietal lobe lesions may cause constructional apraxia
e. The frontal lobes are important in organising and planning sequences of behaviour

2. Match the loss of higher cerebral functions in numbers 1–3 with the most appropriate term from the options given

Options

A. Aphasia   **B.** Apraxia
C. Agnosia   **D.** Parietal
E. Frontal   **F.** Temporal

1. Loss of ability to recognize objects by touch
2. Difficulty executing motor tasks
3. Difficulty speaking, reading and writing
4. The above may be caused by a lesion in which cortex?

3. Loss of fear and emotion is often observed in a lesion in

a. The septal nucleus   **b.** The amygdaloid nuclei
c. The thalamus   **d.** The sensory cortex
e. None of the above

4. The following are functions of the limbic system

a. Olfaction   **b.** Gustation
c. Feeding behaviour   **d.** Sexual behaviour
e. Aggression

EXPLANATION: HIGHER CEREBRAL FUNCTIONS

Higher functions are shared throughout the cerebral cortex and are not confined to a particular lobe. High level cognitive disorders such as **agnosia** and **aphasia** may occur following lesions to the **parietal cortex**. **Wernicke's area** is the cortical area of **language comprehension** (sensory speech) and is located in the **dominant hemisphere**. **Aphasia** is the inability to produce any speech and may occur following damage to either **Wernicke's** or **Broca's** areas. Some brain functions like speech and hand dominance are located in one cerebral hemisphere only. This is known as **cerebral asymmetry** or dominance. The location of the Wernicke's and Broca's areas is shown below: remember 'speak before you think' (the speech motor area is anterior to the speech sensory area).

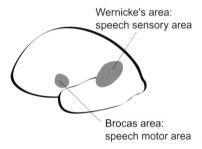

Wernicke's area:
speech sensory area

Brocas area:
speech motor area

'Remember–speak before you think'
(speech motor area is anterior
to speech sensry area)

Most right-handed people are left-sided cerebral dominant. Fifty per cent of left-handed people are left-sided dominant, and 50 per cent right-sided dominant. Ninety per cent of people are right-handed anyway, so it follows that the majority of people have left-sided cerebral dominance. The **frontal lobes** are related to **behaviour**, **planning**, **organization**, **concentration** and **inhibition**.

The **limbic system** is an important collection of anatomical structures in the **medial** aspect of the **temporal lobes**. Important components of the limbic system are the:

- Fornix
- Amygdala
- Parahippocampus
- Septal nuclei
- Cingulate gyrus
- Hippocampus
- Entorhinal cortex

The limbic system is involved in **memory** and **emotion**. The **hippocampus** and **parahippocampal** areas are important in acquiring **new memories**. Damage to the **amygdala** may lead to blunting of emotions – particularly **loss** of **fear**. Other types of behaviour are also influenced by the limbic system including **aggression**, **feeding** behaviour and **sex drive**.

Answers
1. F T F T T
2. 1 – C, 2 – B, 3 – A, 4 – D
3. F T F F F
4. T F T T T

5. Concerning the pharmacology of addiction

A. Explain the concept of 'pharmacological tolerance'

B. Give two examples of compounds which may cause physiological dependence

6. The hypothalamus

a. Influences the autonomic nervous system (ANS)

b. Controls pituitary endocrine functions

c. Is involved in thermoregulation

d. Contains osmoreceptors

e. Has a role in the control of circadian rhythms

7. Loss of circadian rhythm may be caused by damage to which hypothalamic nucleus?

a. Suprachiasmatic

b. Supraoptic

c. Ventromedial

d. Dorsomedial

e. Paraventricular

ADH, antidiuretic hormone; ANS, autonomic nervous system; Ca^{2+}, calcium ion; CNS, central nervous system;

EXPLANATION: PHARMACOLOGY OF ADDICTION

Pharmacological tolerance can be defined as 'the need to progressively **increase** the **dose** of a drug in order to produce the **original desired effect'** (5A).

Tolerance is thought to occur through **increased metabolism** of the drug compound and/or by **neuroadaptive** changes in the CNS such as downregulation of **receptor sites**, an **increase** in Ca^{2+} **channels** and changes in the second messenger system. These changes all reduce the efficacy of a drug, and require an increased dose to have the original desired effect.

There are many compounds that may cause physiological dependence and this is definitely not a finite list, but some examples are: alcohol, nicotine, benzodiazepines (e.g. temazepam, diazepam), cocaine, amphetamines, opioids (e.g. heroin, opium, methadone), caffeine (5B).

EXPLANATION: THE HYPOTHALAMUS

The **hypothalamus** is part of the **diencephalon** and has an important role in **homeostasis** (the control of basic regulatory body functions such as thermoregulation). It controls elements of both the **sympathetic** and **parasympathetic** ANS. It also plays a major role in the control of pituitary hormone release, sending nerve fibres to the **posterior pituitary gland** where it triggers the release of **oxytocin** and **ADH**, and sends releasing hormones into the blood which pass through the pituitary portal system to control release of hormones from the anterior pituitary. The hypothalamus also influences appetite, thirst (hence osmoreceptors) and helps control circadian rhythms via the suprachiasmatic nucleus. Important nuclei of the hypothalamus are shown below.

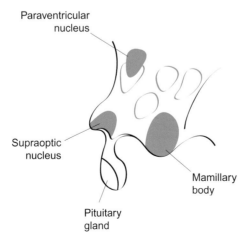

Paraventricular nucleus

Supraoptic nucleus

Mamillary body

Pituitary gland

Answers
5. See explanation
6. T T T T T
7. T F F F F

8. Concerning sleep: REM

    a. Is characterized by delta-waves on electrocardiogram (ECG)
    b. Is a deep and dreamless sleep
    c. Is characterized by paralysis of muscles
    d. Is referred to as paradoxical sleep
    e. Is only seen in sleep walkers

9. A healthy adult has an EEG with the electrodes over the occipital poles. His eyes are closed and he is sitting at rest. What is the most likely EEG rhythm observed?

    a. Alpha
    b. Beta
    c. Delta
    d. Theta
    e. A combination of those above

10. Sleep deprivation

    a. Can cause psychotic episodes
    b. Is associated with sluggishness of thoughts
    c. Increases alertness
    d. Has little effect on an individual
    e. May increase risk of seizures in epileptics

ECG, electrocardiogram; EEG, electroencephalogram; REM, rapid eye movement

EXPLANATION: SLEEP PHYSIOLOGY

Sleep involves a **reduced responsiveness** to environmental stimuli with characteristic **EEG changes**.

EEG recordings from an alert subject record **beta-waves**. **Alpha-waves** are generated if an individual **closes their eyes** and is in a **relaxed** state. There are four stages of sleep, **stage four** is the deepest sleep and is called **'slow wave sleep'**, characterized by delta waves on EEG. Stage four sleep is interrupted by periods of REM sleep with an EEG trace similar to that of someone who is alert – hence it is sometimes referred to as paradoxical sleep.

Answers
8. F F F T F
9. T F F F F
10. T T F F T

11. **Match the symptoms to the psychiatric disorder**

Options

   A. Schizophrenia
   B. Bipolar affective disorder
   C. Anxiety
   D. Obsessive compulsive disorder
   E. None of the above

   1. Mania
   2. Palpitations
   3. Auditory hallucinations
   4. Low mood
   5. Repetitive hand washing

12. **The following are features of schizophrenia**

   a. Hallucinations
   b. Paranoia
   c. Depression
   d. Mania
   e. It may be inherited

13. **In schizophrenia the following neurotransmitter systems are targets for drug treatment**

   a. Acetylcholine (ACh)
   b. Dopamine
   c. Noradrenaline
   d. Glutamate
   e. 5-Hydroxytryptamine (5-HT)

ACh, acetylcholine; 5-HT, 5-hydroxytryptamine (serotonin)

EXPLANATION: PSYCHOTIC DISORDERS

Mental illness is common. One in four of us will suffer from some form of mental illness during our lifetime. One in 100 will acquire schizophrenia.

An individual is said to be **psychotic** if they suffer from: **delusions** (culturally inappropriate fixed ideas and beliefs) and **hallucinations** (reacting to something that isn't actually there – usually visual or auditory but may involve olfaction).

There is a spectrum of psychotic illness – the two most important examples are schizophrenia and bipolar affective disorder.

The key symptoms of **schizophrenia** are: hallucinations, delusions, thought disorders and behavioural disturbances.

Patients with **bipolar affective disorder** may present with similar symptoms to those with schizophrenia, but their mood (also known as 'affect') is also altered – they may alternately suffer from: depression (sadness, low self-esteem, poor appetite) and mania (a euphoric high energy state).

Both bipolar affective disorder and schizophrenia have **genetic components**. It is thought that schizophrenia is caused by overactivity of the mesolimbic projections of the central dopaminergic pathways.

Answers
11. 1 – B, 2 – C, 3 – A, 4 – B, 5 – D
12. T T F F T
13. F T F F F

14. Neuroleptic drugs may cause

a. Decreased dopamine turnover
b. Increased activity in dopaminergic neurons
c. Sleepiness
d. Increased motor activity
e. Increase in prolactin

15. Neuroleptic drugs may cause the following symptoms

a. Increased release of prolactin
b. Lactation
c. Parkinsonism
d. Depression
e. Abnormal facial movements

16. Neuroleptic drugs act on the following receptors

a. gamma-aminobutyric acid (GABA)
b. 5-hydroxytryptamine (5-HT)
c. Histamine
d. Noradrenaline
e. Dopamine

17. The following drugs are atypical neuroleptics

a. Chlorpromazine
b. Ranitidine
c. Haloperidol
d. Risperidone
e. Olanzapine

GABA, gamma-aminobutyric acid, 5-HT, 5-hydroxytryptamine (serotonin)

EXPLANATION: DRUGS USED TO TREAT PSYCHOTIC DISORDERS (THE NEUROLEPTICS)

Drugs used to treat psychoses are called **neuroleptics** – they act on a variety of receptors but **dopamine receptor antagonists** are the mainstay of treatment and target dopamine receptor subtypes D1–D5. Because many of these drugs block dopaminergic receptors, they may mimic the effects of Parkinson's disease – a phenomenon known as 'Parkinsonism'. These drugs normally take around two weeks to start working.

The side-effects of the various classes of neuroleptics are shown below.

Dopamine antagonists	Muscarinic antagonists
Parkinsonism	Dry mouth
Increase prolactin release	Blurred vision
	Constipation

Alpha-adrenoceptor antagonists	Histamine H^1 receptor antagonists
Postural hypotension	Sedation

Newer drugs such as risperidone, clozapine and olanzapine belong to a group of drugs known as '**atypical**' neuroleptics. Their mechanism of action has yet to be fully explained. **Chlorpromazine** and **haloperidol** are older neuroleptics. **Ranitidine** is a **histamine receptor** antagonist, but is not used in psychosis (it is used to reduce acid secretions in the stomach).

18. Write brief notes on depression

A. State four common symptoms

B. Suggest two classes of drugs that may be used in treatment

19. In depression SSRIs are useful because they

a. Block alpha-adrenoceptors

b. Do not cause nausea or headache

c. Do not cause dry mouth or constipation

d. Have a faster speed of onset compared to most antidepressants

e. Often succeed when other antidepressants fail

20. Antidepressant drugs

a. May take several weeks to produce their antidepressant effect

b. Act on 5-hydroxytryptamine (5-HT) or noradrenergic pathways in the central nervous system (CNS)

c. Are useful for preventing suicide

d. May selectively inhibit monamine oxidase (MAO)B

e. Often raise blood pressure

ANS, autonomic nervous system; *BNF, British National Formulary*; CNS, central nervous system; ECT, electroconvulsive therapy; 5-HT, 5-hydroxytryptamine (serotonin); MAO, monoamine oxidase; MAOI, monoamine oxidase inhibitor; SSRI, serotonin selective reuptake inhibitor

EXPLANATION: DEPRESSION

Depression is a **common** psychiatric disorder and has numerous presenting symptoms. The important ones are (18A):

- Sadness (melancholia)
- Loss of motivation
- Anorexia (loss of appetite)
- Loss of interest in people
- Loss of libido
- Early morning waking
- Social withdrawal

Drugs are the most common treatment for depression although psychotherapy is effective and ECT may be reserved for resistant cases. Treatment aims to boost levels of 5-HT and noradrenaline in the brain.

First-line treatment for depression are **SSRIs** (18B) e.g. **fluoxetine**. These drugs prolong the action of serotonin in the synaptic cleft. You can read about them in the *BNF*.

Tricyclic antidepressants (18B) (**imipramine** and **amitriptyline**) are older drugs with more side-effects – especially in the ANS – e.g. dry mouth, blurred vision, constipation. You can read about them in the *BNF*.

MAOIs block the breakdown of noradrenaline after it has been taken back up in to the nerve terminal. These drugs have numerous **side-effects**, e.g. postural hypotension, and people who take them must avoid foods containing **tyramine** (such as wine and cheese) or risk a hypertensive crisis, the so-called '**wine and cheese reaction**'. The selective inhibitor for MAOB avoids many side-effects of the older MAO drugs.

This diagram of a nerve terminal explains the effect of amephetamine on the release of noradrenaline. Amphetamine has a similar structure to noradrenaline and is taken up into the nerve terminal by the noradrenaline transporter, uptake 1. Once inside the nerve terminal it causes widespread release of noradrenaline. While MAO can metabolize noradrenaline, it cannot metabolize amphetamine. Consequently, the action of amphetamine may be prolonged.

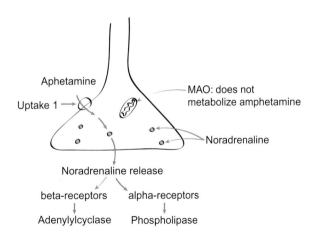

Answers
18. See explanation
19. F F F T T
20. T T T F F

21. Symptoms of anxiety include

    a. Palpitations
    b. Reduced concentration
    c. Cool peripheries
    d. Sweating
    E. Dyskinesia

22. Benzodiazepines

    a. May cause respiratory depression
    b. May cause vivid dreams
    c. Can produce physiological dependence
    d. May be used to treat status epilepticus
    e. May prove useful in reducing the tone of spastic muscles

23. List four effects of diazepam. Draw a diagram showing its mechanism of action

---

Cl^-, chloride ion; 5-HT, 5-hydroxytryptamine (serotonin); GABA, gamma-aminobutyric acid

EXPLANATION: ANXIETY DISORDERS

People with **anxiety disorders** experience symptoms of anxiety out of proportion to a stimulus. Anxiety commonly accompanies **depression**. Symptoms include: **palpitations**, **fearful anticipation**, **poor concentration**, **sweating** and **tremor**.

Psychotherapy and anxiolytic drugs are both treatment options. Drug therapy concentrates on the GABA (important) and 5-HT (less important) neurotransmitter systems. **Benzodiazepines** are effective at reducing symptoms of anxiety quickly. They act via the GABAergic system and have a sedative effect. They may cause **dependence, respiratory depression** and **vivid dreams**.

Benzodiazepines are very useful drugs and, as well as being used as an anxiolytic, may also be used as a **hypnotic, muscle relaxant** and an **anticonvulsant** (23) (in cases of **epilepticus** – a prolonged generalized seizure lasting for more than 30 minutes).

The mechanism of action of diazepam is shown in the figure below (23).

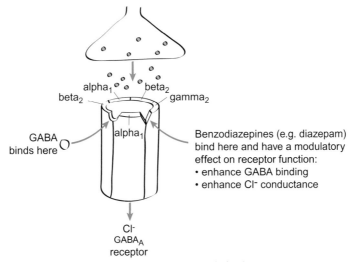

24. Epilepsy

a. Rarely presents in childhood
b. May be cured by surgery
c. May cause loss of consciousness
d. Is related to changes of electrical activity in the brain
e. May be monitored by an electroencephalogram (EEG)

25. Match the symptoms in the numbered list with the most appropriate type of seizure

Options

A. Complex partial seizure
B. Simple partial seizure
C. Absence seizure
D. Generalized seizure
E. Simple partial seizure leading to generalized seizure

1. Loss of consciousness only
2. Tonic–clonic seizure
3. Twitching of muscles in right hand
4. Jerking of the arm and loss of consciousness
5. Jacksonian march

26. The following are drugs used in the treatment of epilepsy

a. Carbamazepine
b. Phenytoin
c. Nifedipine
d. Lamotrigine
e. Vigabatrin

Ca^{2+}, calcium ion; EEG, electroencephalogram

EXPLANATION: EPILEPSY

Epilepsy results from a transient **disturbance in the electrical activity** of the brain with a resulting disturbance in brain function. This manifests as **seizures**, or sometimes **loss of consciousness**.

It commonly presents in childhood and is frequently due to damaged tissue in the brain. In some cases this tissue may be removed **surgically** which may cure the patient. Other causes include faulty Ca^{2+} ion channels (a channelopathy) which may be an inherited condition. Seizures may be monitored by EEG which may be useful in diagnosis of epilepsy. The first-line treatment for epilepsy is pharmacological.

There are two types of epileptic seizure. **Partial seizures** start in a small part of the brain (called a '**focus**') and remain localized. The character of the seizure is related to the brain anatomy. An epileptic focus at A on the figure below would be likely to produce effects in the motor cortex, an example would be involuntary mouth movements. If the patient loses consciousness during the seizure (normally when the temporal lobe is affected), it becomes known as a **complex partial seizure**. **Generalized seizures** occur if the abnormal electrical activity spreads throughout the brain and the whole body may be affected. Many generalized seizures present with rhythmic jerking of the muscles; this is described as a **tonic–clonic** seizure (formerly known as a grand mal seizure).

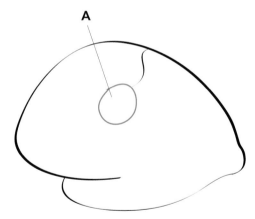

A

Partial seizures may spread to become generalized seizures; the **Jacksonian march** occurs when the seizure starts in the periphery such as a finger and gradually affects more of the body as it moves up the arm to more distant parts.

Answers
24. F T T T T
25. 1 – C, 2 – D, 3 – B, 4 – A, 5 – E
26. T T F T T

27. For each of the drugs below, indicate briefly its mechanism of action in the CNS.

A. Imipramine
B. Phenytoin
C. Vigabatrin
D. Carbamazepine

28. Match the effect with each of the drug groups in the numbered list

Options

A. May cause Parkinson's disease-like symptoms
B. Is metabolized to an active form *in vivo* by a decarboxylase enzyme
C. Enhance the action of gamma-aminobutyric acid (GABA)
D. Cause pinpoint pupils
E. Help prevent suicides

1. Antidepressants
2. Heroin
3. Haloperidol
4. Benzodiazepines
5. L-Dopa (levadopa)

CNS, central nervous system; 5-HT, 5-hydroxytryptamine (serotonin); GABA, gamma-aminobutyric acid; GABA-T, GABA-aminotransferase; Na^+, sodium ion

EXPLANATION: NEUROPHARMACOLOGY

27A. **Imipramine** belongs to the **tricyclic** drug class of **antidepressants**. These compounds have ring structures and work by blocking reuptake of noradrenaline and/or 5-HT. In the case of imipramine, it acts solely by blocking reuptake of noradrenaline. Tricyclic antidepressants are older, but effective drugs. They may have sedative effects and are **dangerous** in **overdose** situations – if the dose is large enough **heart arrhythmias** and sudden death may result. Tricyclic antidepressants are contraindicated in heart disease.

27B. **Phenytoin** is an **antiepileptic** – and acts by **binding** to closed (inactivated) **voltage-gated Na$^+$ channels** preventing them opening. Because normal signals along the neuron result in only a small proportion of Na$^+$ channels becoming inactivated at any one time, the number of channels blocked by phenytoin in a healthy state is insignificant. In an epileptic state with high-frequency repetitive electrical signals, the number of inactivated voltage-gated Na$^+$ channels increases considerably and so does the ability of the drug to block the operation of these channels. Its rate of metabolism varies greatly between individuals, and levels in the plasma must be monitored by **blood tests**.

27C. **Vigabatrin** is another **antiepileptic** drug but acts as an irreversible **inhibitor** of the enzyme **GABA-T**, which is responsible for the breakdown of GABA in the nerve terminal. The inhibition of GABA-T **raises GABA levels** in the brain and the amount of GABA released is also increased. GABA's action as a depressant of the CNS can be exploited by reducing excitability of neurones in patients suffering from epilepsy.

27D. **Carbamazepine** is an **antiepileptic** and provides its therapeutic effects in a similar way to phenytoin, blocking inactivated voltage-gated Na$^+$ channels. Serum concentration of carbamazepine increases in proportion to dose, unlike the unpredictable phenytoin, which makes it a first-line choice in epilepsy.

Answers
27. See explanation
28. 1 – E, 2 – D, 3 – A, 4 – C, 5 – B

29. The following are features of prion diseases

    a. Dementia
    b. Neurodegeneration and astrogliosis
    c. They may be acquired through infection
    d. Slow progression
    e. Long incubation period

30. Multiple sclerosis

    a. Is an infectious disease
    b. Is characterized by an inflammatory process
    c. Has no known cure
    d. Is not a fatal condition
    e. Is characterized by a relapsing remitting course

EXPLANATION: PRION DISEASES

Prions are rod-like **proteins**, they occur naturally in neurons and normally do not cause damage. The pathogenic prion mutant responsible for prion diseases may be **acquired** through **infection** or through a **genetic mutation**. It is protease resistant and anchors to the cell membrane where collections of prions form plaques which lead to **neurodegeneration** and scarring (**astrogliosis**). Examples of prion diseases are **Creutzfeldt-Jacob disease** and **Kuru**.

EXPLANATION: MULTIPLE SCLEROSIS

Multiple sclerosis is a **chronic demyelinating disease**. It is thought to be an autoimmune process where the **oligodendrocytes** are destroyed by **T-cell infiltrates**. It is not an infectious disease. Small patches of myelin are destroyed and cause **temporary localized neurological deficits** such as blindness. Following recovery, further lesions occur, and further **remission** – eventually recovery becomes incomplete and the progress of the disease **becomes more and more severe**. The drug interferon-B helps slow the progress of the disease but there is no cure. It is a **terminal condition**.

31. Memory

    a. Information from different modalities is combined within sensory memory
    b. Unless rehearsed, information held in short-term memory store becomes unavailable after five seconds
    c. Short-term memory capacity is usually less than ten units of information
    d. Superior recall of initial items in a free recall task is due to sensory memory
    e. Neurological deficits of long-term memory may still allow adequate performance in the digit span test

32. Regarding short-term memory

    A. What are the temporal and storage capacity limitations of short-term memory?
    B. How is information lost from the short-term store?

33. Characteristics of Alzheimer's disease include

    a. Intracellular neurofibrillary tangles
    b. Intracellular amyloid plaques
    c. Deranged amyloid protein synthesis
    d. Selective loss of cholinergic neurons
    e. Shrinkage of the lateral ventricles

34. Alzheimer's disease

    a. May be inherited
    b. May feature neurodegeneration caused by glutamate release
    c. Is associated with altered amyloid precursor protein metabolism
    d. Causes ACh levels in the brain to increase
    e. May be caused by a prion-related protein mutation

ACh, acetylcholine

EXPLANATION: MEMORY AND ALZHEIMER'S DISEASE

Information stored in **short-term memory** is typically only held for up **to 20 seconds**, unless it is rehearsed. It is often held in acoustic code which introduces errors into stored information. The short term memory store has only limited capacity – less than a **dozen 'items'**, typically 7 ± 2 numbers. This function is assessed using the **digit span** test **(32A)**.

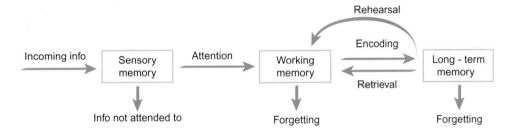

Information is lost from short-term memory in two ways: **displacement** and new attention i.e. new information comes in and old information is replaced, and by **decay factor** – unless information is rehearsed, it degrades as shown in the figure **(32B)**.

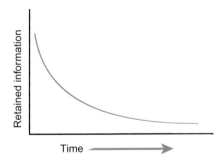

Alzheimer's disease is a form of **dementia** and causes loss **of anterograde memory** (short-term memory) and later, generalized cognitive impairment. **Intracellular neurofibrillary tangles** are present in Alzheimer's and are composed of clumps of microtubules with an abnormal variant of microtubule-associated protein (called tau). **Amyloid plaques** are seen, but they are located extracellularly – this abnormal beta-amyloid arises due to an enzymatic mutation and subsequent error in protein synthesis. **Cholinergic neurons** are lost from the entorhinal cortex and hippocampus early on. Later more generalized cortical loss occurs which results in cortical atrophy and an enlargement of the ventricles. Alzheimer's disease may be inherited.

Answers
31. T F T F T
32. See explanation
33. T F T T F
34. T F T F F

INDEX